DIRECT PAYMENTS AND PERSONAL BUDGETS
Putting personalisation into practice

Jon Glasby and Rosemary Littlechild

Revised and substantially updated third edition

First published in Great Britain in 2016 by

Policy Press
University of Bristol
1-9 Old Park Hill
Bristol BS2 8BB
UK
t: +44 (0)117 954 5940
e: pp-info@bristol.ac.uk
www.policypress.co.uk

North American office:
Policy Press
c/o The University of Chicago Press
1427 East 60th Street
Chicago, IL 60637, USA
t: +1 773 702 7700
f: +1 773-702-9756
e:sales@press.uchicago.edu
www.press.uchicago.edu

ISBN 978-1-4473-2676-2 paperback
ISBN 978-1-4473-2675-5 hardcover
ISBN 978-1-4473-2679-3 ePub
ISBN 978-1-4473-2677-9 Mobi

Cover design by Policy Press
Front cover: image kindly supplied by www.alamy.com
Printed and bound in Great Britain by CMP, Poole
The Policy Press uses environmentally responsible print partners

For Matthew, Mary and Anne-Marie

For John, Hannah, Catriona and Jamie

Contents

List of tables, figures and boxes

Tables

Figures

Boxes

Glossary and authors' note

As explained below, this is a complex area where the key terms can be a source of confusion. As a result, this glossary seeks to provide some basic definitions to simplify subsequent debates as much as possible.

Direct payments: introduced formally under 1996 legislation; the individual receives the cash equivalent of a directly provided service. This was initially available for social care only, and can be used to contract with a private/voluntary sector agency or to become an employer by hiring one's own staff – it cannot be used to purchase public sector services. More recently, direct payments are also available for some forms of health care.

In Control: a national social enterprise, independent from government, which developed the concept of personal budgets and has worked with a number of local authorities around the country to support implementation.[1] In Control's first Chief Executive, Simon Duffy, later left to set up the Centre for Welfare Reform.

Independent living: a key aim of the disabled people's movement has been to achieve independent living (a situation in which disabled people have as much choice and control over their lives as everyone else). This does not mean doing everything oneself – in practice, no one is truly independent; we are all interdependent on others to meet our needs as human beings.

Indirect payments: prior to the Community Care (Direct Payments) Act 1996, many local authorities overcame legal uncertainties by making indirect or third-party payments.

Individual/personal budget: a new way of working pioneered by In Control. At its most simple, it involves being clear with the person from the outset about how much money is available to meet their needs, then allowing them maximum choice over how the money is spent/how much control they want over the money. Initially, the individual budgets developed by In Control were for social care funds only. Subsequently, Department of Health pilots began to explore scope for integrating a series of additional funding sources (and its use of the term 'individual budget' therefore tends to refer to a single pot with the potential to bring together all the various funding available to the individual). After disappointing results from this attempt to integrate funding sources, the term 'personal budget' tends to be

---

[1]   Initially known as 'in Control' (with a lower case 'i'), this organisation later rebranded itself as 'In Control' (with a capital 'I'). For the sake of consistency, the latter is used throughout.

used for approaches involving adult social care funding only. This book follows the policy rhetoric by referring to 'personal budgets' for adult social care funds, and to 'individual budgets' for more integrated sources of funding.

Personalisation: as explained later in this book, official policy has tended to describe a range of ongoing changes in terms of a 'personalisation agenda'. This is rarely clearly defined but is often used as a shorthand for a series of different approaches seeking greater choice and control, tailoring support to individual circumstances, building community capacity and developing a more preventative approach. Opinion is divided as to whether this is a useful shorthand for a broader shift in the nature of service provision or whether it confuses more than it illuminates.

Self-directed support: as explained in Chapter Five, personal budgets are only one part of a new system for social care, which In Control called 'self-directed support'. Some people have found this more helpful than the concept of 'personalisation' and a better way of describing some of the changes covered in this book than by focusing simply on 'personal budgets'.

While we have tried to write a textbook that will be relevant to readers in England, Wales, Scotland and Northern Ireland (and beyond, we hope), some of the specifics of policy and practice guidance tend to refer primarily to England (although we have referred to key statutory instruments from the other countries of the UK wherever possible).

Unfortunately, different surveys of direct payments and personal budgets adopt different definitions, so it is often not possible to make direct comparisons between the data.

Although policy and practice websites frequently change, all relevant internet resources/web addresses were accurate as this book went to press.

In putting together this third edition, we are grateful to Policy Press for all their help and support. While we have included a broad range of sources, we have found work by the following authors particularly helpful and are grateful for their contribution to these debates: Vidhya Alakeson, Peter Beresford, Sarah Carr, Simon Duffy, Caroline Glendinning, Chris Hatton, Jill Manthorpe, Catherine Needham, Martin Routledge and Colin Slasberg.

ONE

Introduction

This introduction provides:

- an overview of the book and its approach;
- an explanation of why the time is right for a third edition;
- a brief note on terminology.

The 1996 Community Care (Direct Payments) Act, which came into force on 1 April 1997, has been described as holding out 'the potential for the most fundamental reorganisation of welfare for half a century' (Oliver and Sapey, 1999, p 175). After long-standing pressure from a range of user groups, the Act empowered social services departments to make cash payments to service users aged between 18 and 65 in lieu of direct service provision. Although progress was initially slow, the number of direct payments has continued to increase and the original Act has been extended to include groups such as older people, younger people aged 16 and 17, carers and the parents of disabled children. As lessons began to emerge from both research and practice, the first edition of this book (*Social work and direct payments*, 2002) sought to provide an introductory textbook to summarise the history and nature of direct payments, promote good practice and explore the implications of direct payments, both for service users and for social work staff.

Since 2002, adult social care has changed almost beyond recognition. Initially discretionary, direct payments quickly became a national performance indicator and began to be compulsory for all local authorities to offer to those who met the criteria (see Chapter Three). They also quickly became associated with the so-called 'modernisation' of adult social care, viewed by policy makers and other key commentators as a core mechanism for changing and improving social care services. From 2003, the concept of a direct payment was supplemented by the notion of a personal budget. Although technically entirely separate from the advent of direct payments, personal budgets nevertheless have much in common with this agenda and seem to offer an even more powerful tool for reforming the system as a whole (see Chapter Five). Under this approach, the local authority gives the person an immediate indication of how much money is available to spend on meeting their needs, and then allows them to choose how this money is spent and how much direct control they have over the money itself. Pioneered initially by a social enterprise known as 'In Control', this way of working was taken up with enthusiasm by the then New Labour government as part of a broader 'personalisation' agenda (HM Government, 2007; DH, 2008a). As our second edition came out in 2009 there were widespread changes taking place at pace and scale, and significant optimism around the impact this might have. However, with hindsight, something important was arguably lost in the process of implementation (a common theme that recurs throughout the history of public service reform more generally) – and this third edition comes at an extremely difficult time in the history and evolution of adult social care and welfare services more generally.

Since the second edition of this book, the personalisation agenda has continued to be a key feature of adult social care, but has also started to spread to other sectors (especially to areas of health care). In future, all adult social care will be delivered via a personal budget (except in an emergency) – and the government has stated that its assumption is that most will receive this via a direct payment. This agenda has been challenging to implement – and has generated significant controversy and debate as front-line practitioners and people using services have struggled to make sense of these ways of working in a very challenging financial and policy context.

Over time, there has also been an increase in the number of new studies exploring the outcomes of personal budgets (a literature which was still very limited back in 2009). In particular, the initial national evaluation of personal budgets (IBSEN) had only just appeared when our second edition went to press (Glendinning et al, 2008), and production was delayed in order to incorporate a brief summary of findings as the research was published. Several years later, there is now greater formal evidence and practical experience around this way of working and the way in which it has been implemented nationally and locally. In particular, Simon Duffy, one of the key architects of personalisation, has asked the question 'Is personalisation dead?' (Duffy, 2012a) and has described what we have in some areas as a form of 'zombie personalisation' (a pale imitation of what true personalisation could and can be) (Duffy, 2014, p 178). These debates are controversial, contested and emotive (see Chapter Six for further discussion; see also Needham and Glasby, 2014) – and the time is right for a third edition that places the continued development of direct payments and the spread of personal budgets in a broader context of austerity and ideological debates about future welfare reform.

Terminology and approach

As non-disabled writers addressing a concept pioneered by disabled people, we follow disabled academics such as Morris (1993a) and Oliver (1990, 1996) in adopting a social model of disability. Whereas medical approaches have tended to focus on the physical limitations of individuals, the social model of disability emphasises the physical and attitudinal barriers that exclude disabled people from participating fully in society (Oliver, 1990). Thus, the focus of intervention should be the current social organisation rather than the individual. Central to the social model is the distinction between two key concepts (Oliver, 1990, p 11):

- *impairment:* lacking part or all of a limb; or having a defective limb, organism or mechanism of the body;
- *disability:* the disadvantage or restriction of activity caused by a contemporary social organisation which takes little or no account of people who have physical impairments and thus excludes them from the mainstream of social activities.

As a result, disabled writers have tended to advocate the use of terms such as 'disabled people' to refer to the oppression that people with impairments experience as a result of prejudice and discrimination:

> People are disabled by society's reaction to impairment; this is why the term disabled people is used, rather than people with disabilities. The latter term really means people with impairments whereas the disability movement prefers to use the politically more powerful term, disabled people, in order to place the emphasis on how society oppresses people with a whole range of impairments. (Morris, 1993a, p x)

In keeping with this approach, we use the term 'disabled people' to refer to all people with an impairment, retaining 'people with physical impairments' as a technical term to distinguish such service users from other user groups (such as people with learning difficulties or people with mental health problems). Thus, the term 'disabled people' is used inclusively to refer to all people with an impairment, whatever their age, whatever the nature of their impairment and whatever category formal services would place the person in.

In addition, it is important for us to be clear from the start about the approach we have taken to many of the issues raised in this book. Having analysed the evidence, talked to disabled people receiving direct payments and personal budgets, worked alongside social care practitioners and engaged with policy makers, we believe that these two ways of working are among the most powerful tools available for increasing the choice and control available to disabled people and for changing the relationship between the state and the individual. While there remain significant barriers to further progress (particularly in a difficult financial and policy context), we believe that many, if not all, of these are to do with the way in which direct payments and personal budgets have been operationalised either nationally or locally, and are not inherent in the concepts themselves. Writing this third edition, we are more pessimistic than we were in 2009 – but we still believe that these concepts and tools can make a massive difference to people's lives, to the job satisfaction of practitioners and to the budgets of hard-pressed public services. Whatever the pros and cons of the current context, these are still the main instruments available, and workers face a choice as to whether to disengage from these discussions altogether – or to try to make these ways of working operate as best they can on behalf of people using services. If we had to choose a sub-title for this third edition – it might be 'we still believe …'

History – why direct payments and personal budgets are different from what went before

This chapter explores:
- the evolution of social care and its relationship with financial issues;
- ongoing pressure for reform;
- the relationship between the state and the individual.

To understand the importance of direct payments and personal budgets, it is necessary to have a basic awareness of the history of social work, its relationship with financial/poverty issues and the traditional relationship between the state and the individual recipient of services. As a result, this chapter provides a brief overview of the origins of modern social work in 19th-century philanthropy and the now notorious Poor Law, the build-up to the Community Care (Direct Payments) Act 1996 and some reflections on the post-war evolution of social care.

Social work and finance/poverty

The Charity Organisation Society

Social work, as a profession, has its origins in 19th-century philanthropy and in the pioneering approach of the Charity Organisation Society (COS) (Bosanquet, 1914; Rooff, 1972; Lewis, 1995). Founded in 1869, COS was essentially a reaction against a proliferation of philanthropic activity following the depression of the late 1860s. By offering charity to the poor, it was argued, the rich were encouraging them to become dependent on alms and exacerbating rather than resolving the problem. For leading COS figures such as Charles Loch or Helen Bosanquet, poverty was caused by individual and moral failings – by fecklessness and thriftlessness. As a result, the solution lay in individual casework, with a COS worker assessing whether an individual was worthy or unworthy of assistance. For those deemed deserving, access to charitable resources might be permitted, although the emphasis was still very much on the need for moral reformation and for the individual to change and improve their ways. For the undeserving, charity should be denied and the applicant left to rely on the harsh mechanism of the Poor Law and the workhouse. Although relatively little is known about the reaction of the poor to this form of charity, it seems likely that many felt aggrieved by this patronising and highly judgemental approach to poverty. Certainly when an East End clergyman and his wife sought to abolish almsgiving and establish a local COS, they were besieged by an angry mob on more than one occasion. In the end, such demonstrations became so widespread that the clergyman had to cut a door from the vicarage to his church so that he could slip out and fetch the police whenever the mob gathered outside (Barnett, 1918, p 84).

The Poor Law

For those deemed undeserving of COS assistance, the only other option was the Poor Law. Associated with legislation from the reign of Elizabeth I, the Poor Law levied poor rates and provided support to those in need via the workhouse and via outdoor relief. As Englander (1998, pp 2–3) explains:

> Outdoor relief … embraced payments for all sorts and conditions – weekly pensions to the aged and infirm, payments for the foster care of village orphans and the upkeep of illegitimate children; casual doles for those in need due to unemployment or sickness; payments for doctor's bills and grants of food, fuel and clothing, particularly during periods of dearth.

Although outdoor relief was technically abolished in 1834, it continued to be paid in practice well into the 20th century (Fraser, 1984; Novak, 1988; Rose, 1988), and was later extended during the 1920s and 1930s to include a complex range of measures to support the poor during the Great Depression (Thane, 1996). Despite this, the Poor Law is most associated with the brutal and dehumanising regime of the workhouse.

To ensure that state support did not encourage the able-bodied to become idle, the 1834 Poor Law Amendment Act promoted the concept of 'less eligibility' (that is, that the workhouse should be made as harsh as possible so that residents were less well off than even the poorest workers outside the workhouse): 'To this end, indoor relief was made as disagreeable as possible by vexatious regulations, want of social amenities, hard labour, poor dietaries and the impact of strict discipline' (Englander, 1998, pp 11–12). Rising at 6am in the summer and 8am in the winter, inmates worked until 6pm, families were separated and distinctive uniforms were enforced to emphasise 'pauper' status and advertise residents' shame (Englander, 1998). Hardly surprisingly, such institutions were bitterly resented by the working classes, many of whom would rather have starved than enter the workhouse (Chinn, 1995). As a result, the 1834 Poor Law Amendment Act was greeted with widespread rioting (Edsall, 1971) and the brutality of the Poor Law has been immortalised by writers such as Charles Dickens (1867).

As unemployment soared in the 1920s and 1930s, new sources of financial assistance were introduced to provide support for the poor (Fraser, 1984). In the 1920s, attempts were made to reduce the cost of such support through the introduction of a stringent 'means test' and a 'genuinely seeking work' test (Thane,

1996). Henceforth, all applicants for state support would have their finances and situations fully assessed, only receiving payments if they were extremely impoverished and if no other source of support was available. Once again, such intrusion into the lives of the poor was heavily resented (Thane, 1996), and the oppressive nature of the system has been widely condemned in literature such as Greenwood's *Love on the dole* (1969).

The abolition of the Poor Law

As pressure mounted to reform the Poor Law, there was a growing awareness that social work should seek to distance itself from its 19th-century origins in order to rid itself of the taint of the Poor Law. Thus, when the Poor Law was finally abolished in 1948, it was replaced by a national scheme for the payment of social security benefits and by new legislation to provide welfare services for older and disabled people. For the first time in its history, social work was separated from the administration of income support and, unlike in most other European countries and the US, social care workers were to play no active part in assessing eligibility for social security payments:

> [The 1948 National Assistance Act] repealed the old Poor Law and replaced it with assistance provided by the National Assistance Board and local authorities. Whereas the Poor Law had dealt with the financial and non-financial welfare of those in need, this Act now divided these up: financial welfare was to be dealt with by the National Assistance Board, whereas it was now the responsibility of local authorities to deal with the non-financial welfare of disabled people, older people and others. Thus, the system developed a sharp separation between cash and in-kind assistance. Social security was to be about the provision of cash, subject to national rules. The social services were to operate locally and apply a much greater degree of discretion in their day-to-day work. This split is not typically found in continental Europe, where local social workers are often involved in the payment of cash benefits. (McKay and Rowlingson, 1999, p 59)

At the time, the separation of social work and social security was seen as a major advance, since social workers would be able to support those in need without the stigma of the old Poor Law (Jordan, 1974). With hindsight, however, the attempt to distance social work from cash payments to those in need has arguably been responsible for practitioners' subsequent failure to address poverty issues. Although the vast majority of people who use social work services are in receipt of social security benefits, many social workers have tended to distance themselves from the material difficulties of their clients and have little 'poverty awareness' (Becker, 1997; p 93; Parrott, 2014), viewing money problems as being the responsibility of other agencies. This contributed to a rapid expansion in specialist money advice services from the early 1970s onwards, often run through voluntary organisations and specialist local authority units rather than through social services departments. Despite a growing awareness of the importance of poverty issues (Becker, 1997; p 93; Parrott, 2014), a change in government funding for specialist advice centres (Cabinet Office, 2012) and some calls for social workers to be more directly involved in the relief of poverty (Mantle and Backwith, 2010), social work has yet to develop a significant anti-poverty perspective (Becker, 1997; Parrott, 2014).

Thus, the desire of the social work profession to distance itself from its 19th-century roots has resulted in a somewhat ambiguous relationship between the profession and cash payments to those in need. Against this background, the introduction of direct payments in 1996 must be seen as a radical departure from previous practice, re-establishing the profession's links to its pre-1948 history. Although direct payments are provided in lieu of services and are therefore very different from outdoor relief or COS charity, the involvement of social workers in making cash payments to disabled people represented a fundamental shift in the nature of the profession, turning the clock back nearly 50 years. This is not only of interest to social historians, but may also help to explain why some social services departments have been slow to take up the opportunities offered by direct payments (see Chapters Three, Four and Eight).

Certainly, concerns about a potential shift in social work practice were prominent in the early 1990s following a number of attempts to introduce a Private Member's Bill to legalise direct payments (see Chapter Three). In response, the health secretary, Virginia Bottomley, wrote to the MP responsible, suggesting that 'social services legislation is concerned with the arrangements of services and not with direct payments, which is the province of the social security system' (quoted in Hatchett, 1991, pp 14–15). Several years later, the issue was to re-emerge following the passage of the Community Care (Direct Payments) Act 1996, with fears that social services departments might be turned into 'income maintenance organisations' and that the Benefits Agency might be considering transferring the administration of certain disability benefits to social services (Hirst, 1997). On other occasions, concerns have been reversed – with suggestions that personal budgets could lead to social care funding being transferred to the social security system (see, for example, Gainsbury, 2008). Although these fears have so far proved groundless, they demonstrate the fundamental shift that has taken place as a result of direct payments, and provided an early indication that the social work profession might not necessarily welcome the new reforms with open arms (see Chapters Four and Eight for further details). In many ways, the development of personal budgets makes these issues even more fundamental, and the cultural challenges of self-directed support are explored in more detail in Chapters Five and Six.

Pressure for direct payments

Following the National Assistance Act 1948, service provision slowly began to evolve away from its initial emphasis on residential care to include a wider range of community services (Means and Smith, 1998a–b; Means et al, 2008). Despite this, pressure for change and for more responsive and flexible services increased, culminating in 1996 with the passage of the Community Care (Direct Payments) Act. The growing body of research in this area suggests that the introduction of direct payments can be traced to three separate but interrelated developments, each of which is reviewed below (Glendinning et al, 2000a, pp 7–9):

- the shortcomings of directly provided services;
- pressure from the Independent Living Movement;
- the experience of the Independent Living Fund.

Directly provided services

Following the 1990 community care reforms, there was ongoing evidence that local authority services were too inflexible and unresponsive to meet the needs of many service users. In 1994, the British Council of Disabled People (BCODP) published the results of research based on interviews with 70 disabled people from four case study local authorities (Zarb and Nadash, 1994). Although the findings of this study are discussed throughout this book, the research highlighted a number of common criticisms, including lack of control, flexibility and reliability (see Box 2.1).

Box 2.1: Disadvantages of directly provided services

1 **Lack of control over times when support is supplied:**
- disrupts day-to-day routines;
- reduces personal freedom;
- is unreliable.

2 **Lack of control over who provides assistance:**
- increases feelings of intrusion on privacy;
- reduces choice over characteristics of support workers (for example, age and gender);
- no sanctions to ensure quality of assistance provided (other than complaints procedures adopted by service providers).

3 **Inability to control type of assistance and how it is provided:**
- leads to inefficiency (for example, workers breaking things, putting household items away in the wrong place, not preparing food to personal tastes);
- increases stress;
- reduces personal dignity and feeling of being in control of one's life.

4 Unreliability:
- increases stress and practical inconvenience;
- reduces ability to control times when assistance is provided;
- can disrupt family life, social life and other activities;
- limited sanctions available if services do not respond to requests for support;
- reduces confidence in support arrangements;
- increases practical demands on other family members.

5 Lack of flexibility:
- can create gaps in assistance provided;
- reduces likelihood of securing back-up and emergency cover for usual sources of support;
- reduces ability to increase support when needs vary;
- can increase vulnerability to breakdown of support arrangements;
- increases reliance on respite services;
- increases reliance on informal support.

6 Interpersonal relationships with staff:
- lack of choice over staff can lead to intrusion on privacy;
- difficulties with changing staff if interpersonal problems arise;
- limited sanctions available if unhappy with attitudes or behaviour of staff;
- larger number of staff to deal with can be inconvenient and/or stressful.

7 Other disadvantages:
- increased vulnerability if service provision reduced or withdrawn;
- uncertainty about future levels of local community care provision;
- concerns about charging and/or means testing.

(Zarb and Nadash, 1994, pp 88–90)

Under the NHS and Community Care Act 1990, social services departments were given a specific brief to target scarce resources on those with the greatest needs (DH, 1990). With regard to domiciliary care, this accelerated the trend towards rebranding traditional 'home help' services as 'home care', focusing on personal care rather than housework and often excluding people with 'low-level' needs (Clark et al, 1998). Such changes were frequently accompanied by an increased tendency to define home care interventions in terms of specific tasks, rather than on an hourly basis, leading to complaints of institutionalisation and of reducing opportunities for more generalised social interaction between care staff and service users (Glendinning et al, 2000a). At the same time, reductions in the length of hospital stays and the emphasis on maximising the throughput of patients resulted in patients being discharged to the community with far greater health needs than would once have been the case (Glasby and Littlechild, 2004). This meant that district nurses increasingly dealt with more complex needs and focused much more on technical nursing care, leaving users with fewer health needs to social services home carers (Barret and Hudson, 1997). Throughout all these changes, there is a growing consensus that care remained service- rather than needs-led, and that both health and social care providers were geared more to crisis intervention than to promoting independence and social inclusion (Morris, 1993a; Glasby and Littlechild, 2004). Perhaps the most striking example of the inflexibility of traditional services comes from Morris's (1993a) description of the experiences of 50 disabled people. This research painted a distressing picture of restrictive services that seek to fit the individual to the service and serve only to increase, rather than reduce, dependency (see Box 2.2). Against this background, direct payments must be seen as a means of enhancing both choice and control, overcoming the traditional limitations of directly provided services.

Box 2.2: Fitting the individual to the service

Marcia's home carers will not assist her with housework or shopping.

Home carers would not assist Mary's husband to have a bath, and the family had to approach their GP to argue that Mary's husband needed a bath for medical reasons.

To get help washing his clothes, William had to argue that this need was created by incontinence.

Catherine's social services department offered to send someone round between 5 and 7 o'clock as this was when they had staff available – even though Catherine did not need assistance at this time.

Elizabeth is Afro-Caribbean and feels that white home carers do not know how to look after her hair properly.

One carer argued with Susan about the way her underwear was placed. Susan tried to deal with this politely, but eventually lost her temper: "Who's fucking wearing it, me or you?"

Vicky feels that the care assistants who visit her are homophobic and do not understand her life.

(Morris, 1993a, ch 7)

Independent living

Although the shortcomings of directly provided services are widely recognised, the most vehement criticisms have often come from the Independent Living Movement. The concept of independent living originated in 1973 in the US, where three disabled students were able to attend university at Berkeley, California, with the support of personal assistants (PAs) provided by the university (Evans,

1993). After graduation, these three students felt that the PA system had been so successful that they established the world's first Centre for Independent Living (CIL), an organisation run and controlled by disabled people, which sought to support other disabled people in taking greater control of their lives and services. Nicknamed the 'quad squad' (since most of the original students were paralysed from the shoulders down), one of the students used an iron lung and went on to become the equivalent of the director of social services in California (Evans, 1993, p 59). Initially, the Berkeley CIL had five key aims, focusing on housing, personal assistance, accessible transport, an accessible environment and peer support. Within ten years, there were 200 CILs in America (Evans, 1993, p 60), and the concept began to spread overseas. In the UK, CILs were founded in Hampshire and in Derbyshire during the early 1980s. Also at this time, the formation of the British Council of Disabled People (established in 1981) and the European Network on Independent Living (ENIL, founded in 1989) provided a national and international focus for the promotion of independent living. More recently, the creation of a National Centre for Independent Living (NCIL) provided further impetus, subsequently merging with other like-minded organisations to form Disability Rights UK. From the beginning, the concept of PAs working under the control of disabled people has been a central feature of independent living, pioneering many of the concepts that were later to form part of the direct payments agenda.

The philosophy of the Independent Living Movement is based on four key assumptions (Morris, 1993a, p 21).

- All human life is of value.
- Anyone, whatever their impairment, is capable of exercising choices.
- People who are disabled by society's reaction to physical, intellectual and sensory impairment and to emotional distress have the right to assert control over their lives.
- Disabled people have the right to participate fully in society.

Although definitions of independent living vary, they all emphasise the importance of choice and control (see Box 2.3) – central features of the Community Care (Direct Payments) Act 1996. As summed up by former NCIL Chief Executive, Frances Hasler: 'Direct payments are a means to an end and that end is independent living. We need to hang on to that. Direct payments are not a good thing or a bad thing in themselves. Direct payments are just a way of getting to independent living' (Hasler, 2000, p 6).

Box 2.3: Independent living

Independent living is the concept of the empowerment of disabled people and their ability to control their own lives.

Independent living is when disabled people live within the community and control the decisions affecting their own lives.

Independent living is a way of choosing and taking control of your own lifestyle. It is all about choosing and controlling what to do, when to do it, and who should do it.

Independent living is a dynamic process. It is about creating choices and identifying solutions. It is a way of life that grows as you grow and develops as you develop.

Independent living is a philosophy and a movement of disabled people who work for equal rights and equal opportunities, self-respect and self-determination. Independent living does not mean that disabled people do not need anybody, that they want to do everything by themselves in isolation. Independent living means that disabled people want the same life opportunities and the same choices in everyday life that their non-disabled brothers and sisters, neighbours and friends take for granted. That includes growing up in their families, going to the neighbourhood school, using the same bus, getting employment that is in line with their education and abilities, having equal access to the same services and establishments of social life, culture and leisure. Most importantly, just like everyone else, disabled people need to be in charge of their own lives, need to think and speak for themselves without interference from others ... In order to reach the same control and the same choices in everyday life that non-disabled persons take for granted a number of prerequisites are necessary. For persons with extensive disabilities there are two key requirements: personal assistance and accessibility in the built environment including accessible housing. Without these two necessities persons with extensive disabilities, in many countries, can only choose between being a burden on their families or living in an institution. These extremely limited and limiting options are incompatible with the concept of independent living.

(NCIL, nda; Ratzka, nd)

The Independent Living Fund

Prior to the introduction of direct payments, the Independent Living Fund (ILF) gave disabled people the opportunity to receive cash payments in order to purchase personal assistance. In 1986, the Social Security Act announced measures to replace Supplementary Benefit with Income Support. Whereas recipients of Supplementary Benefit could receive additional payments on the basis of ill-health or disability, the new Income Support would replace such additions with flat-rate disability and severe disability premiums, with much stricter eligibility criteria (Hudson, 1988, 1994). Contemporary estimates suggested that some disabled people would be as much as £50 per week worse off, and there were fears that some of these people would be forced into residential care (Hudson, 1988; Kestenbaum, 1993a).

In response, disability groups began a sustained lobbying process, eventually succeeding in persuading the then Conservative government to make alternative arrangements for those affected by the 1986 Act. After consulting with representatives of disability groups, Nicholas Scott, minister for social security and the disabled, announced details of a new independent trust fund (the ILF) in early 1988 (Kestenbaum, 1993a). Established for a maximum of five years with an initial budget of £5 million, the ILF would make payments to a small number of disabled people who had to pay for personal assistance. The number of applicants was expected to be 'in the hundreds rather than the thousands' (quoted in Hudson, 1988, p 708), and the Fund was available only to those disabled people on low incomes who had to pay for personal care.

From the beginning, it quickly became apparent that the government had significantly underestimated the demand for the ILF. Although it was initially anticipated that there would be around 300 new awards each year, applications reached the rate of 900 per month in 1989–90 and, by November 1992, 2,000 per month (Kestenbaum, 1993a, pp 29–33). By 1993, some 22,000 people were receiving payments (Zarb and Nadash, 1994, p 6) and the Fund had an annual budget of £82 million (Kestenbaum, 1993a, p 32).

As Kestenbaum observed:

> For many applicants, the ILF was not just about making up for unavailable statutory services. It was the preferred option. From a disabled person's point of view, the provision of cash makes the important difference between having one's personal life controlled by others and exercising choices and control for oneself. Money has enabled ILF clients ... not only to avoid going into residential care, but also to determine for themselves the help they require and how and when they want it to be provided. (1993a, p 35)

Research carried out by the ILF suggested that the popularity of this new form of support was largely due to the enhanced choice and control that it enabled (Kestenbaum, 1993b). Drawing on semi-structured interviews with ILF recipients and a large-scale postal questionnaire, Kestenbaum concluded:

> The findings from this research challenge the assumption that disabled people are incapable of exercising effective choice and control over their own care arrangements ... The experience of ILF clients ... shows how, with enough money to have care assistance under their own control, or that of a chosen advocate, many disabled people can greatly improve the quality of their lives as well as stay out of residential care. (1993b, p 78)

Perhaps inevitably, the success of the ILF posed both financial and political problems for the government (Morris, 1993a, p 14). While the Fund had uncovered the need for cash payments to enable disabled people to purchase their own care, the cost was escalating rapidly and local authorities (the lead agencies under the community care reforms introduced in 1993) were prohibited from making such payments (see Chapter Three for further details). After tightening eligibility criteria in 1990 and 1992 and introducing an age limit on the Fund (excluding those aged 75 and over), the ultimate response of the government was to terminate the original ILF, and to replace it with two successor bodies (Hudson, 1993; ILF, 2000):

- the Independent Living (Extension) Fund would continue to administer payments to recipients of the original ILF, although awards were not linked to inflation;
- the Independent Living (1993) Fund would accept new applications but on a different basis. Henceforth, disabled people receiving at least £200 worth of services per week from their local authority could receive a maximum of £375 from the Fund. Crucially, the new Fund was to be restricted to people aged under 66 at the time of their application (see Kestenbaum, 1999, appendix A and ILF, 2000 for eligibility criteria).

Thus, from April 1993, local authority social services departments were responsible for purchasing services to meet the assessed needs of disabled people, using the new ILF to 'top up' existing care packages. This was widely interpreted as a retrograde step that emphasised professional control rather than user-led services and independent living (see, for example, Hudson, 1993; Morris, 1993b). Despite this, the experience of the ILF revealed a number of significant issues that were to influence the subsequent development of direct payments:

- A number of prominent cases raised the need for adequate support systems to ensure that disabled people purchasing their own care were able to meet their legal and financial obligations. In some cases, ILF recipients were left in thousands of pounds of debt, having failed to make National Insurance and other contributions, serving as a powerful reminder of the need to focus on the technicalities of being an employer (Bond, 1996).
- Some disabled people found it very difficult to recruit PAs, and valued support in this area (Kestenbaum, 1993b, pp 12–13).
- Concerns were expressed that any payments to disabled people should take additional costs such as recruitment, employers' contributions and other overheads fully into account (Bond, 1996).
- Some ILF recipients were nervous about what would happen when the community care reforms were introduced, and feared that they could lose their payments (Kestenbaum, 1993b, p 41). During the late 1990s, similar issues were to be raised following the tendency of many local authorities to introduce

direct payments on a pilot basis, leaving some service users unsure whether or not pilot projects would become part of mainstream service provision (see Chapters Three and Four).

• The ILF revealed the potential conflicts that can arise between the aims of the Independent Living Movement and the desire of central government to limit public expenditure (see Chapter Eight for further details).

Above all, however, the ILF enabled disabled people to purchase their own care and represented a fundamental shift in power between professionals and users. As Hudson has commented:

> The ILF offered precisely what many people wanted – a major weekly cash payment … direct to claimants to buy the support they felt they required. For the first time in Britain, users were calling the shots in the purchase and provision of care … In a major and unintended way, the 1986 Social Security Act produced a visionary glimpse of the reality and feasibility of user-led care packages. (1993, p 28)

This was not the original aim of the government, and Morris (1993a, p 13) uses the phrase 'progress by default' to describe how a small-scale government policy measure could have such significant implications for the Independent Living Movement. Indeed, Hudson (1993, p.28) described the ILF as a form of 'Pandora's box' that, once opened, would be very difficult to close again.

While the ILF continued to evolve, its underlying approach remained similar from 1993 onwards and, in 2006, the Department for Work and Pensions commissioned an independent review (Henwood and Hudson, 2007a). This described the ILF as 'an organisation created in haste to solve a particular political problem at a particular point in time' (para 12.4), but gave it credit for having 'played a significant part in the short history of independent living' (para 12.37). The review recommended that the ILF should continue to be administered in its current form for the short term, but that it should ultimately be fully incorporated into the personal budgets programme (see Chapter Five).

In December 2010 the minister for disabled people, in the newly formed Coalition government, declared that the ILF was permanently closed to new applicants. In December 2012 the government made a decision to close the ILF by March 2015 for current recipients (who by then numbered 19,136) and to integrate the support into mainstream care systems administered by local authorities in England and to devolved administrations in Scotland and Wales. Despite a legal challenge by two severely disabled ILF recipients under the Equality Act, the closure was deemed lawful. This was overturned by the Court of Appeal in November 2013 but, following the government's equality analysis (in which it acknowledged that recipients *may* end up receiving less money overall but could equally receive more services directly from their local authority), the government finally confirmed in March 2014 that the ILF would close on 30 June 2015 (DWP, 2014).

On 1 July 2015, £262 million was transferred to English local authorities and the devolved administrations. In England the money is not ring-fenced and there is no obligation on local authorities to support existing ILF recipients to the same extent. In contrast, the Scottish Government has set up a new Scottish ILF to support existing ILF recipients which will be open to new applications. The Scottish ILF will also administer payments to recipients in Northern Ireland. The Welsh Government is allocating a special grant to local authorities to support people on the current scheme until March 2016 when it will be subject to the next spending round. While the exact impact of the closure of the ILF will not be known for some time, recipients are concerned that, despite the introduction of national eligibility criteria for support through the Care Act 2014, their allocation of funding to support independent living may once again become a 'post-code lottery' (Donovan, 2014).

Post-war evolution of social care

This brief overview is illustrative of a more general change in the relationship between the individual and the state that has evolved in British post-war welfare services. In 1948 the National Assistance Act imposed upon local authorities the duty to provide residential care for those people who, by virtue of 'their age, infirmity or any other circumstances are in need of care and attention which is not otherwise available to them'. The care needs of people living in their own homes were then largely met by voluntary organisations and individuals' families and friends, although the role of local authorities in providing community-based services began to extend during the 1950s and 1960s (Means et al, 2008). Nevertheless, the relationship between the state and the individual was largely based on paternalism, with welfare professionals offering assistance from a limited range of prescribed services and characterising people in need of help as passive recipients of care (Audit Commission, 1992). During the 1970s and 1980s increasing concerns about the cost and quality of residential care resulted in a shift of resources from residential to community-based services. At the same time the Conservative government, with Margaret Thatcher as prime minister, made it clear that it saw a reduced role for the state in the provision of social care and an increased need for individual responsibility. Thus, as the 1981 White Paper, *Growing Older*, suggested: 'care in the community must necessarily mean by the community' (DHSS, 1981, p 3).

Although the community care reforms of the 1990s often adopted the rhetoric of citizenship, many of the detailed changes fell far short of a rights-based approach to social welfare (Rummery, 2006). Instead, the emphasis was more on introducing notions of consumerism into welfare policies, with people who used social care services recast as 'customers' with the ability to exercise influence and choice over decisions about their care (DH, 1989). Ultimately, if people using services did not like what they were receiving, the reforms implied that they had the right to take their 'custom' elsewhere. However, as Chapter Eight suggests, many commentators are critical of consumerism, claiming that its application to the majority of people who receive social care services is inappropriate and misplaced (see, for example, Barnes and Walker, 1996; M. Barnes, 1997; Rummery, 2006; Means et al, 2008).

With the election of New Labour in 1997, the 'modernisation' of public services sought 'to deliver efficient, high quality and responsive public services' (Butcher, 2002, p 184), based increasingly around the 'principle of "person-centredness"' (Scourfield, 2007, p 110). While New Labour's 'third way' included a mix of different approaches to reform, the use of markets remained a key strand. More recently, the discourse of the market and consumerism has also featured strongly in the policies of the Coalition government, which, on coming to power in 2010, stated in *A Vision for Adult Social Care* (DH, 2010a, p 15), that 'people, not service providers or systems, should hold the choice and control about their care'. Commentators continue to debate the extent to which the modernisation agenda of these two governments differs significantly from what went before. Certainly, many would argue that the experiences described in Boxes 2.1 and 2.2 above remain just as recognisable now as then. While the focus was less on institutional forms of care and more on intensive support at home, services often seemed just as inflexible and unresponsive as the previous system (see, for example, Raynes et al, 2001; CSCI, 2006). More recent research on older people's experiences of home care services indicates some greater level of choice and control over the flexibility of support offered (Rodrigues and Glendinning, 2014), but still a significant 'gap between the "ideal" of user choice and control and the "reality" of practices' (Rabiee and Glendinning, 2014, p 212).

Chapter Seven addresses in detail how the introduction of direct payments and personal budgets has addressed some of these issues. It documents the largely positive messages that have come from the recipients of direct payments and personal budgets (see Leece and Bornat, 2006, for example, for various accounts of the experiences of direct payment recipients). Nevertheless, difficulties and barriers to implementation still exist, not least of which are some of the tensions experienced by social workers whose role it is to assess people's eligibility for direct payments.

In a study of social workers' approaches to direct payments, Ellis (2007) found that Lipsky's (1980) theory of 'street-level bureaucracy' is still pertinent to the way in which social workers ration their time and resources and act as gatekeepers to direct payments. Ellis (2007, p 409) explains:

> Social workers also face conflict between their legal obligations to ration access to direct payments and their ethical obligation to value self-determination and empowerment – a tension heightened by the rooting of eligibility criteria in functional and financial definitions of independence rather than on autonomy and full participation.

These issues are explored in more detail in Chapter Eight, but here lies the nub of what Duffy (2005a) sees as one of the key limitations of direct payments: that they are still administered within what he calls 'the professional gift relationship' (see also Figure 5.1, Chapter Five). As Waters and Duffy (2007, p 8) maintain:

> Both these approaches [direct payments and the ILF] were still expected to fit within an overall system of Social Care that was not designed to support Independent Living. Although there has been significant progress in moving away from its institutional legacy the assumptions of the past still influence the current system. Today the current system of Social Care is still not designed to treat recipients as citizens who are entitled to support and who can be expected to take control over their own support. Instead support is treated as a 'gift' which is given to people on the basis of an assessment of their needs.

In short, despite the significant changes that have taken place in the design and delivery of services, the underlying ethos of social care and the relationship between the state and the individual have remained remarkably stable over time. In contrast to the professional gift model, Duffy (2005a) advocates a system of self-directed support, based upon citizen entitlement rather than on discretion. These concepts are explored in detail in Chapter Five, but the emerging evidence suggests that self-directed support and personal budgets may address some of the unanswered questions about direct payments – introducing a more even-handed and transparent relationship between the individual and the state, which will address concerns about equity and social justice (Riddell et al, 2005; Rummery, 2006; Ellis, 2007; Scourfield, 2007). However, these issues are contentious – and success is by no means guaranteed. As Waters and Duffy (2007, p 13) caution:

> The approach is a form of co-production – with the [personal budget] forming one part of the new 'contract' between the citizen and the state. However, this shift is not merely technological. It is primarily cultural and it would be wrong to conceive of the cultural change being merely about changes in how professionals think and behave. Self-directed support is a challenge not just to professionals but to the whole of society.

SUMMARY

In order to overcome the stigma of the Poor Law, post-war social work in Britain has been characterised by the separation of social security and social services, with the former focusing on financial needs and the latter on providing welfare services for frail and disabled people. Once widely hailed as a step forward, this separation has since been criticised for enforcing an artificial distinction that does not adequately reflect people's needs, and for depriving social work of an awareness of poverty issues. Against this background, the decision to enable local authorities to make cash payments in lieu of directly provided services represents a major cultural shift that significantly alters the role of social services departments. As a result, those seeking to promote direct payments need to be aware of the magnitude of the task ahead of them in seeking to overcome social workers' opposition to this new way of working (see Chapter Eight for further discussion).

Prior to the introduction of direct payments in 1996, pressure for reform had been mounting for some time. Crucially, key figures in the campaign for change were disabled people themselves, critiquing local authority services, organising themselves into an Independent Living Movement and persuading the government to introduce the ILF. As criticisms of directly provided services increased, the experience of receiving ILF payments began to alter the relationship between service users and service providers, demonstrating the liberating and empowering potential of disabled people's purchasing personal assistance directly. Although the government acted in order to limit the scope of the ILF, services could not return to the pre-1988 situation and reform of some description was almost inevitable.

In post-war Britain there have been a number of minor changes and developments in the relationship between the state and people who use welfare services. A largely paternalistic philosophy has gradually been replaced by one that, at least in principle, acknowledges that people want choice and flexibility in the services they receive. However, people using services – even when they can access a direct payment – still remain recipients of a 'professional gift' without necessarily feeling that they are entitled to support as citizens. Against this background, the advent of personal budgets, discussed in further detail in Chapter Five, has the potential to change fundamentally the relationship between the individual and the state – and it is for this reason that the issues discussed in this book are so contentious but also so important.

IMPLICATIONS FOR POLICY AND PRACTICE

- Historically, social workers held an important role in administering cash payments to people in need of financial help. However, the advent of the post-war welfare state meant this was removed when a national system for the payment of social security benefits was established.
- As direct payments are now mandatory in all local authorities and as personal budgets are introduced, social work practice must once again be prepared to engage with financial issues.

- Central to direct payments and personal budgets are the principles of independent living. Some social care professionals may find these challenging to their current practice and so be reluctant to advocate for direct payments and personal budgets.
- The introduction of direct payments and personal budgets represents a fundamental change in the relationship between the state and the individual (which will have implications for service users, families, practitioners, managers and policy makers alike).

RECOMMENDED READING AND USEFUL WEBSITES

For those interested in the historical overview provided above, Payne (2005) offers an interesting account of the origins of social work, with a comprehensive list of references and relevant websites.

Accessible accounts of the development of post-war social care services can also be found in Glasby (2012a), Glasby and Littlechild (2004), Means and Smith (1998b) and Means et al (2008).

Morris (1993a) gives an overview of the philosophy of the Independent Living Movement and summarises accounts from disabled people about the inflexibility of directly provided services.

Henwood and Hudson's (2007a) review of the Independent Living Fund can be accessed via www.melaniehenwood.com/perch/resources/fullilfreport.pdf, while the government's equality analysis of the closure of the ILF can be found at https://www.gov.uk/government/uploads/system/uploads/attachment_data/file/287236/closure-of-ilf-equality-analysis.pdf.

Parrott (2014) gives a detailed overview of the relationship between social workers and financial issues and their role in combatting poverty.

Butcher (2002) explores the concept of citizenship, while Rummery (2006) looks specifically at the role of direct payments in supporting disabled people to become full citizens.

A number of commentators take a more critical look at the role of direct payments and personal budgets in addressing issues of social exclusion, including Ellis (2007), Riddell et al (2005), Rummery (2006), Ferguson (2007) and Scourfield (2007). Many of the issues raised here are explored in further detail in Chapters Seven and Eight of this book.

A key player in the campaign for direct payments was the National Centre for Independent Living, which has since merged with other like-minded organisations to form Disability Rights UK (http://disabilityrightsuk.org). For historical and grey literature, the Disability Archive (http://disability-studies.leeds.ac.uk/library/) is an excellent resource (including for a number of hard-to-access but crucial accounts of the history of the independent living movement.)

For personal budgets, access the In Control website (www.in-control.org.uk) and that of the Centre for Welfare Reform (http://www.centreforwelfarereform.org).

REFLECTIVE EXERCISES

1. For current practitioners and students, to what extent are you familiar with the history of social work? How does this help you to reflect on the relationship with financial issues and to put the development of direct payments/personal budgets in a broader context?

2. To what extent are you fully 'independent' as you go about living your life, and to what extent do you feel interdependent on others? To what extent would adult social care support you to live a life of your choosing if you were using services?

3. Reflecting on the critique of directly provided services in Box 2.1, to what extent have we solved these problems – or are they still current/common?

4. Thinking about other aspects of your life, what balance do we strike between the state and the individual in different walks of life? To what extent has adult social care kept up with changes in this broader relationship? What opportunities might direct payments/personal budgets offer to revisit these issues?

THREE

Direct payments – where they came from and how they developed

This chapter explores:
- indirect payments and the campaign for direct payments;
- the Community Care (Direct Payments) Act 1996;
- the extension of direct payments and recent policy developments.

Despite the growth of the Independent Living Movement and the popularity of the ILF, direct payments to individual service users were illegal under Section 29 of the National Assistance Act 1948 until the passage of the Community Care (Direct Payments) Act 1996. Although the Social Work (Scotland) Act 1968 did permit direct payments in certain circumstances, these were heavily prescribed and the power to make such payments was rarely used (Zarb and Nadash, 1994; Witcher et al, 2000). Nevertheless, pressure had begun to build for some sort of cash payment to enable disabled people to make their own care arrangements (see Chapter Two). Against this background, this chapter covers the key milestones in the campaign for direct payments, from the growth of indirect payments in the 1980s–1990s to their place within the personalisation agenda of the 21st century.

Indirect payments and the campaign for direct payments

As awareness about the potential advantages of enabling disabled people to purchase their own care increased, both service users and local authorities began to explore methods of circumventing the prohibitions of the National Assistance Act. For John Evans, then chair of the BCODP Independent Living Committee, it was crucial to get rid of 'that damn silly law from 1948, and accept that direct payments for some people are just common sense' (quoted in George, 1994, p 15). Others agreed, and a range of schemes were developed in different parts of the country to make payments to disabled people, some of doubtful legality (Mandelstam, 1999). Although arrangements varied, the two main approaches were to make payments via a third party (such as a voluntary agency) or via an independent trust (see Box 3.1 for examples).

Probably the first example of indirect payments was in Hampshire in the early 1980s, where a group of disabled people were able to move out of residential care after persuading their local authority to take the pioneering step of making payments to each individual via the original residential home (Project 81, nd; Shearer, 1984; Zarb and Nadash, 1994, pp 5–6; Brindle, 2008). Although the

Hampshire scheme faced closure because of legal concerns raised by the county's solicitor and treasurer, a report from the Audit Commission (1986, p 69) cited Hampshire's payment scheme as an example of innovative good practice (Evans and Hasler, 1996). This proved enough to save the project, and Hampshire remained a key player during the implementation of direct payments.

Box 3.1: Indirect payments

To overcome legal restrictions, Lauren used to receive payments from her local authority via a housing association. This meant that the housing association was the employer, not Lauren. So she took further action to enhance her control of her care package. On the suggestion of a friend, Lauren set up a trust to receive the payments on her behalf. The trust deed was drawn up by a solicitor, and Lauren served as a trustee together with three friends. Lauren now employs four PAs and is able to work and care for her mother. To ensure accountability to the local authority, a social worker sits on the trust.

(Morris, 1993a, p 122)

One example is that of Lothian Social Work Department who, having assessed someone's personal assistance needs, makes a quarterly cash payment in advance for the cost of paying for that assistance to the Edinburgh Voluntary Organisation Council. The payment is passed on to the individual who then uses it to either employ their own personal assistants, or to employ agency staff.

(Morris, 1995)

Over time, payment schemes began to expand and, in 1990, research commissioned by RADAR found that 59% of 69 participating local authorities made payments to disabled people, either directly or indirectly through intermediaries (Browne, 1990, quoted in Hatchett, 1991, p 14). The latter included charities, housing associations and national organisations such as the Spinal Injuries Association (Hatchett, 1991, p 14; Craig, 1992, p 47; Morris, 1993a, p 26). Although payment recipients were often individuals who had taken the initiative in putting their case to the local authority (Morris, 1993a), most participating authorities in the study suggested that they would welcome legislation enabling them to make such payments (Craig, 1992, p 47).

In 1994, researchers from the Policy Studies Institute (PSI) carried out a national survey of local authorities in England, Wales and Scotland, with a 64% response rate (Zarb and Nadash, 1994). The study found that just under 60% of participating authorities were already operating payments schemes (most of which involved indirect payments through a third party or through trusts). This figure was almost identical to the RADAR study of 1990, the key difference being that there was far less evidence in the 1994 survey of authorities making payments directly to service users than in 1990 (5% and 23% respectively). However, this was felt to be a product of contemporary legal concerns, following government statements on the illegality of direct payments (to be discussed later). As a result, several authorities had taken legal advice, changed from direct to indirect payments or ceased making payments altogether. Despite this, just over 90% of respondents indicated that they would make direct payments if legislation permitted, with only three authorities stating that they were definitely opposed to such changes.

Thwarted reforms

As evidence of the benefits of paying cash sums to individual service users increased, so pressure began to mount for legislation to promote direct payments. Throughout this process, organisations of disabled people and advocates of independent living were at the forefront of the campaign for change, lobbying Members of Parliament, organising meetings and commissioning research (Evans and Hasler, 1996). A good example of the way in which disabled people were able to take the lead in the campaign for direct payments comes from Kingston-upon-Thames, where an early and prominent payments scheme was established on the initiative of two local disabled people. As part of this process, the disabled people approached the social services department with their proposal for a payments scheme, produced formal documentation for the social services committee and participated in a pilot scheme (Macfarlane, 1990; DH, 1998a).

As part of the lobbying process, BCODP quickly found an influential supporter in Andrew Rowe, Conservative MP for Faversham and mid-Kent (Evans and Hasler, 1996). Having encountered the concept of direct payments through a disabled member of his constituency, Rowe became a committed supporter of the Independent Living Movement and was a key player in campaigning for the legislative changes which were finally introduced under the Community Care (Direct Payments) Act 1996. During parliamentary debates on the NHS and Community Care Bill in 1990, the issue of direct payments was raised in both the House of Commons and the House of Lords, with a number of proposed amendments to promote direct payments. Unfortunately, this campaign was to backfire, with serious and unintended consequences. Having examined the issue of making cash payments to disabled people, the government found that this practice was illegal under the National Assistance Act and, in the policy guidance accompanying the community care reforms, reminded local authorities that current legislation 'prohibit[ed] the making of cash payments in place of arranging services' (DH, 1990, p 26). Thus, a measure designed to promote the concept of direct payments and support existing payment schemes had actually resulted in such schemes being declared illegal (personal communication, Andrew Rowe). This was to cause considerable difficulties for a number of local authorities, who were broadly supportive of direct payments yet understandably concerned to operate within the law.

Once direct payments had been declared illegal, the only course of action was to campaign for new legislation to overturn this prohibition. In 1992, Andrew Rowe tried to introduce a Private Member's Bill (the Disabled Persons (Services) Bill), which would have enabled disabled people who were able and willing to do so to employ their own staff, with the bills paid by the local authority. While Andrew Rowe's preferred choice was for disabled people to control their own payments, his Bill was designed to overcome considerable Treasury concerns about the danger of public money being misappropriated (personal communication). The Bill failed to become law, with key concerns about the perceived difficulty of establishing adequate procedures to ensure that public money was spent appropriately and the possible risk that PAs might exploit or abuse disabled people (Zarb and Nadash, 1994; Campbell, 1996).

Throughout the events described above, considerable lobbying and campaigning was taking place, without much apparent success. While groups of disabled people met key politicians who appeared to support independent living schemes, campaigners perceived that a significant barrier to support for a change in legislation was the government's concern that direct payments schemes would cost too much (Evans and Hasler, 1996). In response, the BCODP Independent Living Committee decided to change its tactics somewhat, commissioning independent research in order to investigate the cost implications and effectiveness of direct payment schemes. With funding from the Joseph Rowntree Foundation (JRF), BCODP was able to commission the PSI to undertake the desired research. The resulting study, *Cashing in on independence* (Zarb and Nadash, 1994), was a key document and is still referred to time and time again throughout this book and other literature on direct payments. While it is difficult to gauge how successful it was in persuading the government to implement direct payments, it must undoubtedly have been a factor in the government's eventual change of heart on the direct payments issue (to be discussed below).

Despite government opposition to direct payments and the defeat of Andrew Rowe's proposed legislation, the BCODP campaign received significant support from other bodies, most notably from the Association of Directors of Social Services (ADSS) (Evans and Hasler, 1996). In 1992, ADSS adopted a resolution in support of direct payments and became an increasingly active member of the campaign for a change in the law (Taylor, 1996a). In addition to writing the foreword to *Cashing in on independence* (Zarb and Nadash, 1994), Roy Taylor (then chair of the ADSS Disabilities Committee) was a key player in the struggle for direct payments (see, for example, Taylor, 1994, 1995, 1996a–c, 1997). In addition to the ADSS, other key supporters of direct payments included the Audit Commission, the Prince of Wales Advisory Group on Disability, the British Association of Social Workers and the Association of Metropolitan Authorities (*Hansard*, House of Lords Debates 21 April 1993, col 1642; Evans, 2000). Also at this time, the concept of direct payments received qualified support from the House of Commons Health Committee (1993), which felt that more research was required before direct payments could be implemented, but that such payments were consistent with the emphasis of the community care reforms on user involvement and choice.

Despite widespread support for direct payments, some disabled people remained concerned as to what the future might hold with regard to independent living. With the legality of payment schemes thrown into doubt and a series of abortive attempts to introduce new legislation, many disabled people were unsure about the future availability of payments (Zarb and Nadash, 1994). This uncertainty was later to continue after the implementation of the Community Care (Direct Payments) Act1996, for the initial discretionary nature of the reforms meant that disabled people had no guarantees that the various direct payment schemes that had been piloted would continue and be adopted into mainstream service provision. In many ways, this was similar to events in the early 1990s, when the introduction of the community care reforms led to fears about the longer-term availability of ILF payments. There are also parallels with the more recent situation, where some have viewed the introduction of personal budgets as a potential threat to direct payments (see Chapter Five).

Nevertheless, the government was faced with a considerable dilemma as pressure from influential quarters mounted for change. Members of the government had expressed their support for the concept of independent living, and the rationale for direct payments was in line with the principles of choice and control that underpinned their community care reforms. However, there were also concerns about rapidly rising public expenditure and fears about what might happen if direct payments were introduced. In many ways, this combination of commitment to the underlying principles and concerns about the practical and financial implications has also greeted the advent of personal budgets (see Chapter Five).

The Community Care (Direct Payments) Act 1996

The legislation

In November 1994, the government announced its intention to legislate in order to enable local authorities to make direct payments to service users rather than providing community care services directly:

> I [Virginia Bottomley, health secretary] intend to take … a new power to enable social services authorities and social work departments to make direct cash payments to disabled people in lieu of community care services. Direct payments … will give disabled people greater independence and choice and involve them and their carers more fully in their own care. (DH, 1994, p 1)

While it may never be entirely clear what led to this change of heart, there appear to have been a number of key considerations. The imminent launch of the BCODP/PSI research into direct payments (which showed that direct payments were both cheaper than directly provided services and resulted in higher-quality services) may have been a key factor in persuading the government to reconsider its previous opposition (Zarb and Nadash, 1994; Evans and Hasler, 1996). For Andrew Rowe, direct payments were the result of a dedicated and sustained campaign for reform and the momentum for change was simply too strong for the government to resist. Ultimately, 'direct payments were an idea whose time had long since come' (Andrew Rowe, personal communication).

Once the decision had been taken to introduce direct payments, a number of practical matters needed to be resolved before new legislation could be drawn up. As a result, a Technical Advisory Group (TAG), including representatives from central government, local authorities and organisations of disabled people, met to consider some of the technical issues that implementation would raise, drew up guidance for government ministers and civil servants, and contributed to a 1996 consultation paper on direct payments. Although the group included three disability organisations, only one member of TAG was a personal assistance user running her own direct payment scheme (Evans and Hasler, 1996).

Building on the work of TAG, the Department of Health introduced a consultation paper in January 1996 on its proposals for direct payments (DH/Scottish Office/Welsh Office/Northern Ireland Office, 1996). In addition to setting out how direct payments would operate, the consultation paper sought views on a number of key issues to be contained within the regulations and guidance. Central to the government's view of how direct payments should function was the belief that recipients must be 'willing' to receive payments instead of services and 'able' to manage them (DH/Scottish Office/Welsh Office/Northern Ireland Office, 1996, p 3). While service users could receive extensive support from others, they would ultimately remain responsible for the management of their payments.

Crucially, the Direct Payments Bill would give the secretary of state the power to specify which groups could receive direct payments, a move justified in terms of the need to restrict the number of direct payment recipients while the scheme was in its infancy (DH/Scottish Office/Welsh Office/Northern Ireland Office, 1996, pp 3–4). As a result, the consultation paper set out six possible groups of people who might be able to benefit from direct payments, emphasising that its own preference was to limit direct payments to people with physical impairments under the age of 65 (DH/Scottish Office/Welsh Office/Northern Ireland Office, 1996, pp 4–5). While this preference was never enacted, it does give an early insight into official thinking and undoubtedly affected the take-up of direct payments by some user groups (see Chapter Four). Another key issue in the consultation paper was a restriction on using direct payments to employ partners or close relatives (to be discussed later; see also Chapter Eight). This was justified by a desire to prevent existing informal care arrangements from becoming too formalised, to prevent the risk of exploitation and to prevent family members from feeling under pressure to give up their jobs and become full-time carers (DH/Scottish Office/Welsh Office/Northern Ireland Office, 1996, p 8). However, a more cynical interpretation might be that it would prove too expensive to pay family carers for work that they had previously been expected to carry out free of charge as part of their family obligations.

As a result of the government's determination to reserve the power to restrict eligibility for direct payments, the Community Care (Direct Payments) Act 1996 was relatively concise, with the bulk of detail provided through accompanying regulations and subsequent policy and practice guidance. As the government had already indicated in its 1996 consultation paper, the user groups eligible for direct payments could be expanded at a later stage if the experiment proved successful, without the need for further legislation. Consequently, the Act itself simply authorised local authorities to make payments directly to disabled people (see Box 3.2), with the bulk of the reforms to be set out in much greater detail by the secretary of state.

Box 3.2: Key changes under the Community Care (Direct Payments) Act 1996

- Local authorities had the *power*, not the *duty* to provide direct payments.
- Direct payments could be paid to all adult user groups under the age of 65.
- Payments were not to be used for more than four weeks' residential care in any period of 12 months.
- Payments could not be used to employ certain types of relatives and household members.

Thanks to ongoing lobbying by disabled people's organisations, the government's original intention to exclude people with learning difficulties and/or with mental health problems from direct payments was defeated and direct payments were to be available to all adult user groups under 65.

Policy and practice guidance

After the passage of the Community Care (Direct Payments) Act 1996, official policy and practice guidance was issued in May 1997 (DH, 1997; see also DHSSPS, 1997; National Assembly for Wales, 1997; Scottish Office, 1997). In the event, implementation in Northern Ireland was delayed for one year until 1998. However, since 1997/98, the original guidance has been revised and updated as direct payments legislation has been extended and as emerging practice has revealed ongoing barriers to further progress (see, for example, DH, 2000, 2001a–c, 2003a, 2009). Whereas the 1997 policy guidance set out *what* local authorities should do if they chose to exercise their new power to make direct payments, the practice guidance advised on *how* authorities might implement the Act. From the very beginning, the policy guidance emphasised that the government's aim was to enhance the independence of service users by giving them control over the way that community care services are delivered. To maximise this independence, local authorities should work in partnership with disabled people and leave as much choice as possible in the hands of the service user, while at the same time ensuring that the individual's needs are being met and that public money is being used appropriately and cost-effectively. Although authorities now had the *power* to make direct payments, this was not a *duty*, and local authorities retained discretion over whether or not to implement direct payments and the detail of how to do so. However, whatever an authority decided to do, the guidance was clear that it should not treat direct payment recipients any more, or less, favourably than people receiving services, and should continue to develop other ways of making services more responsive.

Since payments were to be made only by local authority social services departments in lieu of community care services, the Act did not allow any other body (such as a health or housing authority) to make direct payments, nor provide for direct payments to be used for health- or housing-related services. Although direct payments could be used for all community care services, this excluded permanent residential care (including a total of more than four weeks' respite care in any 12-month period) and services provided directly by the local authority. Since direct payments are an alternative to community care services, the guidance made it clear that authorities offering payments needed to do so within their existing budgets and should only make a direct payment if this would be at least as cost-effective as the services that would otherwise be arranged.

The original legislation prevented payments to people under 18 or to adults wishing to purchase services for people aged under 18. Although users could ask carers, or other third parties, to help them manage direct payments, the user had to remain in control of the payment and was accountable for the way the money was used. The local authority had to be satisfied that the user consented to receiving payments and understood the financial and legal implications of receiving direct payments (in shorthand, being 'willing and able'). Throughout ongoing debates, it was often restated that payments are designed to enhance independence, not to transfer dependence from a local authority to a third party.

Initially, direct payments were to be made available only to disabled people under 65 (including people with physical impairments, learning difficulties, mental health problems and HIV/AIDS), although people receiving such payments before the age of 65 could carry on receiving them after that age. However, this was to be reviewed after the Act had been in force for one year. In addition, direct payments could not be offered to certain people in the mental health or criminal justice system. The original guidance confirmed that direct payments could not be used to purchase services from a partner or a close relative living in the same household. In addition, services could not be purchased from a close relative living elsewhere or from someone else living in the same household, although authorities could make an exception to this rule if this was the only appropriate way of securing the relevant services. For the purposes of the Act, a close relative was defined as a parent, parent–in–law, aunt, uncle, grandparent, son, daughter, son-in-law, daughter-in-law, step-son or step-daughter, brother, sister or the spouse or partner of any of the above. This restriction has since been revised (see later in this chapter and Chapter Eight for further discussion) and was not meant to prevent disabled people from employing live-in PAs, but to prevent recipients employing people with whom they had a personal, rather than a contractual, relationship.

Drawing on the experience of existing independent living schemes, the practice guidance emphasised that service users are well placed to judge how best to use direct payments and have a vested interest in using their payments properly on necessary services. The guidance acknowledged that direct payments can be complex, but stated that 'the aim should be to set up simple but effective systems, which contain safeguards but are not unnecessarily bureaucratic or time-consuming' (DH, 1997, p 26). Since direct payments are intended to enhance control, this process should begin at the very start through consultations with people with different types of impairment, people from different ethnic backgrounds and people of different ages. In particular, the practice guidance emphasised the importance of adequate support mechanisms, both before an assessment and at the point of making a decision about direct payments. This might include access to someone with employment expertise, a payroll service, lists of local agencies, assistance with drafting advertisements, job descriptions and contracts, rooms for interviewing, training, advocacy or written materials (see Chapter Eight for further discussion of the importance of support services). In particular:

> The experience of users on existing independent living schemes is that they find it easier to seek advice from someone who is independent of the local authority ... People who have experience of managing direct payments themselves are well placed to advise and help others as they begin to receive direct payments. In many areas, people who are managing their own care meet regularly to support one another and to discuss any difficulties which have arisen. This can be an effective way of sharing experience. (DH, 1997, pp 39–40)

The extension of direct payments

When direct payments were implemented in April 1997, policy and practice guidance emphasised that the reforms would be reviewed after one year, with a view to reconsidering the user groups eligible for direct payments (DH, 1997). Although direct payments were introduced by a Conservative government, they received whole-hearted support from the incoming New Labour government in 1997 and continued to do so throughout its term of office (see Box 3.3). In 2003, Stephen Ladyman, then the community care minister, argued that:

The assumption should be not only will care be delivered by a direct payment; the assumption should be that the person can manage a direct payment and the only times when care should be delivered, in my view, other than by a direct payment, is when the individual themselves has made a personal and positive choice to receive the care directly and not via a direct payment. (NCIL, 2003)

Box 3.3: Key policy documents supporting direct payments in England (see also Chapter Five)

Improving the Life Chances of Disabled People (Prime Minister's Strategy Unit, 2005): in this wide-ranging strategy document, the government identified direct payments as a key mechanism for promoting independent living for disabled people.

Independence, Well-being and Choice (DH, 2005): one of the key proposals in this Green Paper was 'wider use of direct payments and individual budgets to stimulate the development of modern services delivered in the way people want' (DH, 2005, para 13.2).

Our Health, Our Care, Our Say (DH, 2006): this White Paper confirmed the government's commitment to expanding direct payments and extending them to groups of people who had previously not been eligible to receive them.

Putting People First (HM Government, 2007): this concordat, produced by central and local government, professional bodies, social care providers and regulators, pledged to increase the number of people receiving direct payments and to roll out personal budgets throughout all adult social care.

The Health and Social Care Act 2008 extended direct payments to people who lack capacity by enabling a direct payment to be made to a 'suitable person' acting on their behalf.

A Vision for Adult Social Care 2010 (DH, 2010a) recognised the importance of direct payments within the wider personalisation agenda.

The Care Act 2014 confirmed the role of direct payments as a crucial means by which people are helped to exercise choice and control over their care.

Since the original 1996 Act, a number of developments have taken place:

- the extension of direct payments to older people, carers, people with parental responsibility for disabled children and disabled young people;
- revised policy and practice guidance;
- changes in legislation to make direct payments mandatory;

- the introduction of a performance indicator on direct payments in 2003 (subsequently abolished in 2010);
- new forms of support to help people access direct payments;
- a change in legislation to allow people who lack capacity and some people subject to mental health legislation to receive direct payments.

On 1 February 2000, new regulations removed the age limit that had initially applied to direct payments, enabling people aged 65 and over to benefit from such payments in authorities that decided to take advantage of the new powers available to them (Age Concern, 2000; Statutory Instrument (SI) 2000/11; see also Scottish Statutory Instrument (SSI) 2000/183; SI 2000/1868 (W127); Statutory Rule 2000/114). Since the original legislation, some policy and practice developments have taken place in Wales and Northern Ireland at a later date than in England but the basic principles have remained largely the same. In Scotland, however, there have been significant similarities, but also some key differences (which are addressed briefly later in this chapter and in Chapter Six – see also Box 3.4).

Box 3.4: Key developments in Scottish legislation and policy

- The Social Work (Scotland) Act 1968 permitted cash payments in exceptional circumstances.
- The Community Care (Direct Payments) Act 1996 enabled payments to adults aged 18–64.
- 2000 – direct payments extended to older people.
- The Community Care and Health (Scotland) Act 2002 placed a mandatory duty on local authorities to offer direct payments from June 2003.
- Accompanying regulations (SSI 2003/243) specified that direct payments were to be offered to parents with parental responsibility for disabled children but, unlike in England, Wales and Northern Ireland, not to carers.
- In contrast to other parts of the UK, the Act extended direct payments to *all* people assessed as having care needs, including people who are 'frail, receiving rehabilitation after an accident or operation, fleeing domestic violence, refugees, homeless or recovering from drug or alcohol dependence' (Pearson, 2006, p 36). The date for this change was subsequently revised from 2004 to 2005 (SSI 2005/114).
- Unlike the rest of the UK, the 2003 regulations also extended direct payments to attorneys and guardians for people unable to manage their own payments.
- Under the 2003 regulations, close relatives who lived with a person receiving a direct payment could not be paid but relatives living elsewhere were eligible for payment. However, the Adult Support and Protection (Scotland) Act 2007, section 63, empowered local authorities 'to offer increased flexibility in tailoring individualised self-directed support packages'. The 2007 regulations (SSI 2007/458) changed the rules on employing close relatives and gave local authorities the discretion to allow a close relative to be employed 'if the local authority is satisfied that securing a service from that person is necessary to meet the beneficiary's need for a service, or that securing a service from such a person is necessary to safeguard or promote the welfare of a child in need' (Scottish Executive, 2007, Section 5, p 111).

- In 2007 the Scottish Executive issued *National Guidance on Self-Directed Support* (Scottish Executive, 2007), building on direct payments legislation, followed in 2010 by *Self-Directed Support: a National Strategy for Scotland* (Scottish Government, 2010). The term 'self-directed support' is often used interchangeably with 'direct payments' (Scottish Executive, 2007, Annex A) but it describes a wider debate about 'the ways in which individuals and families can have informed choice about the way support is provided to them' (Scottish Government, 2010, p 67).
- The Social Care (Self-Directed Support) (Scotland) Act 2013 identified direct payments as one of four options for receiving self-directed support; the others are 'directing the available support' (having a greater say in directing the support without full responsibility), 'arranged services' and a mixture of all three options.

In 2000, the Department of Health issued revised guidance to take account of the relatively slow progress to date in implementing direct payments and the recent extension of the scheme to older people (DH, 2000; see also National Assembly for Wales, 2000; DHSSPS, 2000a–b; Scottish Executive, 2000). Although the guidance was very similar to its predecessor, there were a number of changes in emphasis that seemed to indicate the government's intention to increase the availability of direct payments and to ensure that particular groups of service users were not excluded. As a result, the guidance stressed from the beginning that direct payments have a very broad potential, improving quality of life, promoting independence, aiding social inclusion and encompassing areas such as rehabilitation, education, leisure and employment. The government was clear that it wanted 'to see more extensive use made of direct payments' (DH, 2000, p 3) and that authorities would need to consider how to include people with different types of impairment, people from different ethnic backgrounds and people of different ages. When deciding whether or not to offer direct payments to an individual, authorities should not 'fetter their discretion' (that is, they should consider each case on its merits, even where the authority was not currently offering direct payments, and treat all adult client groups equitably) (DH, 2000, p 4). Although direct payments could still only be offered if they were at least as cost-effective as direct services, there was a recognition that any consideration of cost-effectiveness should consider long-term best value.

At the same time as it issued revised guidance, the government also indicated its intention to introduce legislation to extend direct payments to a range of groups originally excluded from the 1996 Act. The Carers and Disabled Children Act 2000, accompanied by a raft of policy and practice guidance (DH, 2001a–e), empowered local authorities to make direct payments to:

- carers aged 16 and over (for services that meet their own assessed needs to support them in their caring role);

- people with parental responsibility for disabled children (for services to meet the assessed needs of the disabled child or to provide short-term breaks that meet the needs of both parent and child);
- young disabled people (aged 16 and 17).

While the extension of direct payments to carers was broadly welcomed by many commentators, a number of concerns were raised. Disability organisations, such as NCIL (2000), suggested that there was scope for conflict between users and carers, arguing that extending direct payments to other groups should not undermine the basic goal of increasing users' independence. At the same time, some academic commentators adopted a more critical stance to direct payments, outlining some of the inherent political tensions in such schemes and expressing concerns about inequity and the potential social exclusion of some service users (see for example, Scourfield, 2005a, 2007; Spandler, 2004). These issues have now been subsumed within a wider critique of the implementation of personalisation more generally and are discussed in more detail in Chapter Eight.

Nevertheless, the government remained committed to extending the take-up of direct payments and in 2001 made this way of working mandatory rather than discretionary. Under section 57 of the Health and Social Care Act 2001, local authorities must offer direct payments to anyone who is eligible for community care services, consents to receiving payments and is able to do so. Shortly after this extension of direct payments came into effect in 2003, moreover, direct payments became one of the Social Services Performance Assessment Framework Indicators (DH, 2003b). Despite these positive attempts to promote direct payments, however, an unfortunate backwards step came when the Department for Work and Pensions caused widespread confusion with a national campaign to promote its own version of 'direct payments' (social security benefits paid direct into recipients' bank accounts; see CSCI, 2004; DH, 2005).

To accompany legislative changes under the Health and Social Care Act 2001, the government produced new guidance in 2003–04 (DH, 2003a; see also Scottish Executive, 2003; DHSSPS, 2004; Welsh Assembly Government, 2004). Now that direct payments were mandatory, the government recognised that 'for some staff/ professionals, direct payments may require a significant change from current ways of working with people needing services' and that this may involve a 'cultural leap' (DH, 2003a, p 5). While the principles of direct payments remained largely the same as in previous guidance, there were three areas in the 2003 guidance that received additional attention.

- *The employment of close relatives*: a key change was a relaxation of rules about employing close relatives. While direct payments may not ordinarily be used to pay for services from a close relative living in the *same* household, the restrictions were lifted on employing relatives who lived *elsewhere*.
- *Issues of cost-efficiency*: in deciding whether or not direct payments represent a cost-effective option, local authorities can consider long-term issues such

as whether or not direct payments are likely to prevent a future hospital or residential care admission (DH, 2003a, para 87). As in 2000, this was a much wider definition of cost-efficiency than in the original guidance and includes not only social services expenditure, but also possible savings to the system as a whole (see also Chapter Six for further discussion of personal health budgets).

- *Additional support*: in an attempt to encourage new groups of people to receive direct payments and increase the overall numbers of recipients, the Department of Health launched a £9 million Direct Payments Development Fund (DPDF) in 2003, available over three years. The Fund was used to pay for voluntary organisations, in partnership with local authorities, to set up additional information and support services. The DPDF also made a single grant to NCIL, as the key national organisation for disabled people, of £280,000 per year over three years, which included an evaluation of all the projects receiving DPDF funding. In addition, the DPDF was subject to an external evaluation by the Personal Social Services Research Unit (PSSRU) at the London School of Economics, which assessed whether or not the Fund had reached its primary objective of increasing take-up and whether the process of involving the voluntary sector in the grant allocated had worked (Hasler, 2006, pp 150–1). More limited resources for support organisations to perform similar roles were also made available for Scotland, Wales and Northern Ireland (Pearson, 2006).

Building on the issue of appropriate support, findings from the NCIL evaluation (2006) showed that the DPDF helped to increase the number of people receiving direct payments and to get direct payments onto local agendas. During the course of the project an additional 8,483 people received direct payments, twice as many as had originally been estimated (NCIL, 2006, p 12). Box 3.5 gives a summary of some of the key factors that the study found can enhance the take-up of direct payments. Despite this, a national survey of support organisations (Davey et al, 2007a) showed a steady increase in the level of support for direct payments recipients across the UK, but a wide variation in the kind of support available. The survey found that over 50% of people receiving direct payments did not receive help from a support scheme, but it was not clear whether this was because they felt they did not need assistance, found help elsewhere or could not access a support scheme (Davey et al, 2007a, p 92). In England, approximately one-third of support schemes did not provide support to all user groups (which raised concerns that a number of user groups might be missing out on accessing appropriate support). A further concern was about the sustainability of support services, given that the DPDF was time limited. In addition, the survey found that most schemes focused on promoting the take-up and setting up of direct payments, with approximately one-third leaving the maintenance and ongoing management of direct payments to the recipient (which may account for some of the variability in take-up rates between different user groups in Chapter Four). Similarly, in 2002, the Scottish Executive allocated a development grant of £530,000 over two years to Direct Payments Scotland in order to set up user-led support organisations, provide training, build confidence, promote awareness of direct payments at local and national levels and facilitate information sharing (Scottish Executive, 2001).

> **Box 3.5: Factors likely to enhance the take-up of direct payments**
> The evaluation of the DPDF has confirmed that the take-up of direct payments is enhanced if:
>
> - Sufficient levels of consistent support are provided to individual service users.
> - There is good knowledge of direct payments among local statutory organisations and voluntary and community groups.
> - Local authorities take a strategic lead on direct payments.
> - Users are involved in all areas of direct payments.
> - There is understanding of the principles of independent living.
>
> (NCIL, 2006, p 84)

The availability of direct payments was further extended in England by the Health and Social Care Act 2008. Until then, a key anomaly was experienced by parents receiving a direct payment for a disabled child. If the child was assessed as lacking capacity to manage a direct payment when they became an adult, the family/individual should technically lose their direct payment. In the 2006 White Paper, *Our Health, Our Care, Our Say*, the government therefore agreed to extend the availability of direct payments to people who lack capacity, as defined under the Mental Capacity Act 2005, and so are unable to give consent to receiving a direct payment (DH, 2006). In 2008, the Health and Social Care Act extended the availability of direct payments to such people by enabling a direct payment to be made to a 'suitable person' acting on behalf of the person lacking capacity. In addition to benefiting young disabled adults when they become 18, this change may also benefit some adults with head injuries and people with dementia.

The government therefore issued new guidance in 2009 to accompany the legislative changes introduced by the Health and Social Act 2008 (DH, 2009; see also Welsh Assembly Government 2011). Local authorities were now required to extend the offer of direct payments to:

- people who lack the capacity to consent, following the appointment of a 'suitable person' to manage the payment (DH, 2009, pp 65–72);
- most people who are subject to mental health legislation (with some exceptions) (DH, 2009, pp 73–4); people subject to some criminal justice legislation are still excluded from receiving direct payments (DH, 2009, p 97).

The advent of the Conservative-led Coalition government in 2010 continued to focus attention on direct payments as a crucial part of the agenda for the personalisation of adult social care services. One key principle outlined in an early document, *A Vision for Adult Social Care*, stated:

> Individuals not institutions take control of their care. Personal budgets, preferably as direct payments, are provided to all eligible people. Information about care and support is available for all local people, regardless of whether or not they fund their own care. (DH, 2010a, p 8)

This desire to see more direct payments is discussed in more detail in Chapter Six in the context of personal budgets. However, despite the Coalition government's support for direct payments, within months of coming to office, it scrapped the direct payments Performance Assessment Framework Indicator when the local government secretary, Eric Pickles, announced:

> And instead of the National Indicator Set, and instead of every single department's endless demands that you measure this, that or the other, there's just going to be one list of every bit of data that government needs. (DCLG, 2010)

A further change to direct payments followed swiftly. Following the recommendation of the Law Commission (2011), the Care and Support White paper *Caring for our Future: Reforming Care and Support* (HM Government, 2012) declared an intention to extend direct payments to people in residential care. Twenty-two local authorities were recruited into a 'Trailblazer programme' and an independent evaluation was commissioned from the Policy Innovation Research Unit (Ettelt et al, 2013). A scoping study of the use of cash payments to people in residential care in the UK and elsewhere showed limited evidence of effectiveness or cost-effectiveness, and the findings from the relatively small pilot study of 18 local authorities were not conclusive (Ettelt et al, 2015). Nonetheless, the government has stated that by April 2016 all councils must offer direct payments to all eligible people living in residential care.

Following the review of adult social care law by the Law Commission in 2011 (Law Commission, 2011), the Coalition government passed legislation proclaimed by Norman Lamb, then care and support minister, as 'the most significant reform of care and support in more than 60 years, putting people and their carers in control of their care and support' (DH and the Right Hon Norman Lamb, 2014). Implemented in April 2015, the Care Act 2014 has at its centre the principle of person-centred care, which includes local authorities' responsibility for ensuring their citizens' 'well-being'. Sections 31–33 outline the new legislative framework for local authorities to provide direct payments to people with and without capacity. The Care and Support Statutory Guidance (DH 2014a) confirms that:

> Local authorities should aim to develop a range of means to enable anyone to make good use of direct payments and where people choose

other options, should ensure local practice that maximises choice and control. (DH, 2014a, 11.35)

In addition, the 2014 guidance introduces a new element to the payment of family members that:

> allow[s] local authority discretion to give prior consent to pay a close family member living in the same household to provide management and/or administrative support to the direct payment holder. (DH, 2014a, 12.35 p 171)

This does not change the regulations about family members living in the same household being paid only in exceptional circumstances, and is not intended to 'replace the normal family bonds associated with caring' (DH, 2014a, p 171), but recognises the complex administrative task that accompanies substantial direct payments.

Similar legislation was passed in Scotland (the Social Care (Self-Directed Support) (Scotland) Act 2013) and Wales (the Social Services and Wellbeing (Wales) Act 2014), accompanied by statutory guidance (The Scottish Government, 2014a) and draft guidance (Welsh Government, 2014). While direct payments have now become part of a much wider programme of the reform of social care in the UK, they remain an important means by which people receive care and support from the state. The remaining chapters in this book show they have developed in the 20 years since their inception in 1996/97 and their current role in self-directed support.

SUMMARY

After a long and sustained campaign, disabled people were ultimately successful in bringing about the introduction of direct payments. Almost more than any other area of policy and practice, this is a way of working developed by disabled people, lobbied for and promoted by disabled people, and made to work by disabled people. This alone makes the introduction of direct payments a critical policy milestone in adult social care. Since their formal introduction in 1996/97, moreover, their progress has been rapid. Although initially small in terms of overall numbers, direct payments spread to a range of new user groups and have been promoted with enthusiasm by New Labour, the Coalition government and the 2015 Conservative government. Despite the more recent 'personalisation' agenda (see Chapters Five and Six), direct payments continue to be an important means by which care and support services are delivered to people within the UK, and Chapter Four explores the potentially radical impact they have had on services, on staff and on people's lives.

IMPLICATIONS FOR POLICY AND PRACTICE

- Direct payments are an example of a policy that has been developed *by* disabled people *for* disabled people.
- As direct payments have developed since 1997, some of the initial restrictions in their implementation have been removed and developments are ongoing. From the very beginning, they have been promoted enthusiastically by all governments of whatever political persuasion and remain a key feature of adult social care.
- A practical consequence of their rapid growth is that everyone working in social care will need to keep up to date with developments, ensuring that we do not set disabled people up to fail by not informing them of the options available to them.
- The expectations surrounding direct payments were so significant that a degree of disappointment was probably always likely as the practical barriers to change became apparent. However, our contention is that the majority of such barriers are to do with the way in which direct payments were operationalised – not to do with the concept itself (see Chapters Seven and Eight for further discussion).

RECOMMENDED READING AND USEFUL WEBSITES

For background reading on direct payments, see the following:

- Leece is a qualified social worker and practice teacher and has written short and accessible summaries of some of the early key national debates on direct payments and about key practice/implementation issues at a local level (see, for example, Leece and Leece, 2006; Leece, 2000, 2002, 2003, 2004, 2006a–b, 2010).
- This includes an edited collection (Leece and Bornat, 2006), with a series of leading commentators providing contributions on the early experience of different user groups, voices of experience, the implementation of direct payments, workforce implications and future developments.
- The introduction of Gardner's (2014) book *Personalisation in social work* gives an accessible account of the role of direct payments in the context of the personalisation agenda.
- For those who want to place the development of direct payments in a broader context, Perri 6's (2003) article on the history of consumerism and choice in British public services provides a critical overview of developments in education, housing and health and social care.
- Moffatt et al's (2012) article discusses the concepts of choice and consumerism for older people in England and Wales, while Manthorpe et al (2015a) provide a comprehensive overview of the development of self-directed support in Scotland.
- For further detail on how previous boundaries between 'cash' and 'care' are changing, Glendinning and Kemp's (2006) edited collection provides an overview of key national and international developments, including a number of chapters on the implications of direct payments.

More details on the legislation, policy and practice guidance on direct payments in the four countries of the UK can be found in key publications at the following websites:

- www.local.gov.uk/care-support-reform (general context of current social care reforms);
- www.dh.gov.uk (England);
- www.thinklocalactpersonal.org.uk (England);
- www.dhsspsni.gov.uk/directpayments-about (Northern Ireland);
- www.gov.scot and www.selfdirectedsupportscotland.org.uk/ (Scotland);
- http://gov.wales/topics/health/socialcare/directpayments/?lang=en (Wales).

REFLECTIVE EXERCISES

1. There seem to have been a number of underlying factors at work in the campaign for direct payments. To what extent do these feel compatible – or might they subsequently take the reform agenda in a different direction?
2. If you were the secretary of state of the day, how much risk would you have been prepared to accept – and what restrictions/safeguards might you have insisted on if called upon to introduce direct payments?
3. Reflecting on some of the early policy guidance, what impact do you think some of the initial restrictions might have had on the subsequent development of direct payments? (You may wish to reflect again on this question after reading other chapters in this book.)
4. How does the campaign for direct payments compare with other social care reforms? Does the history of direct payments influence how you think about them now and their prospects for the future?
5. Think about those early campaigners – how might they have felt at different stages in the events described in this chapter? Looking back at their contribution, what do you think their legacy might be?

FOUR

The lessons of direct payments – how they spread and what they achieved

This chapter explores:
- the spread of direct payments;
- take-up of direct payments by different user groups;
- international perspectives on direct payments.

Although the passage of the Community Care (Direct Payments) Act 1996 was a major victory for disabled campaigners, the legislation was initially permissive rather than mandatory (see Chapter Three). It was therefore perhaps inevitable that while some authorities would choose to implement direct payments almost immediately, others would be more cautious and possibly even hostile. This has resulted in a situation where the rate of implementation has been uneven both across the UK and between different user groups. Even though direct payments are now mandatory, major barriers still remain. Against this background, this chapter reviews the pace of implementation and the experiences of different user groups, highlighting key obstacles to progress. With the advent of personal budgets (see Chapters Five and Six), much of the more recent literature on the uptake of direct payments effectively conflates these two ways of working. However, where discrete data is available it is presented here. For comparative purposes, brief reference is also made to the international literature in order to summarise emerging lessons from how other cash-for-care systems operate.

The spread of direct payments

Early days

As noted in Chapter Three, research carried out by the PSI two years prior to the Community Care (Direct Payments) Act suggested that many authorities were already making payments to service users and that many more would do so if legislation permitted. Despite this, there were considerable regional variations, with availability generally much lower in the north and the west of Britain compared to the south and London, where 80% of councils were making payments (Zarb and Nadash, 1994, p 27). Overall, the only exception to the concentration of payment schemes in the South was Scotland, where 64% of local authorities were making payments (albeit with low numbers overall) and where such payments had been legal in exceptional circumstances for some time (see Chapter Three).

Immediately after the 1996 Act, progress was not as rapid as Zarb and Nadash's (1994) initial research might have suggested. In 1997, the PSI and NCIL published preliminary findings from a research study into the implementation and management of direct payments (Zarb et al, 1997). Based on a survey of all UK local authorities and on more detailed consultations with ten selected Councils, the research suggested that only 48% of local authorities were operating some form of payments scheme, with about one-third unsure whether to introduce such payments in the future. Although London, the south-west and Scotland had been relatively proactive, provision was very low in the north of England and in Wales and non-existent in Northern Ireland (where implementation was delayed until 1998; Zarb et al, 1997, p 3). This was consistent with the findings of other early studies (see for example, Auld, 1999; Fruin, 2000). In 2000, ADSS surveyed all 171 social services departments in England and Wales, with a response rate of 100% (Jones, 2000). This study found that 80% of authorities had introduced direct payment schemes and that all bar one of the remaining 20% planned to follow suit. Despite this, strong regional variations remained, with direct payments most prominent in London and the south. Around 3,500 people were then receiving direct payments, although a number of authorities had excluded people with mental health problems and/or learning difficulties from their schemes. It was also clear from this research that there were a number of individual authorities that heavily influenced the national overview. For example, Hampshire alone had 400 people receiving direct payments (approximately 11% of all recipients in England and Wales at that time).

In Scotland, the Scottish Executive commissioned a key study on the early implementation of direct payments that identified considerable confusion among local authorities about what direct payments were and how they operated (Witcher et al, 2000). Only 13 (less than half the authorities in Scotland) were making direct payments to a total of 143 people, the majority of whom had a physical or sensory impairment. There were no recipients with mental health problems and no users from a minority ethnic group. While most authorities were positive about the principles of direct payments, the main barriers to implementation included considerable variation in the form and scope of support schemes, lack of flexibility between budgets, variations in payments to individuals and difficulty in recruiting PAs in most authorities, particularly in rural areas (Witcher et al, 2000).In Northern Ireland, with no history of third-party payments (Campbell, nd), initial progress was slower than in other parts of the UK. According to one commentator, the delay was because 'disabled people have shown little interest and health and social services boards are not ready' (Valios, 1997, p 3) – although which one of these perceived barriers may have caused the other remains an important issue to consider.

Elsewhere, it was suggested that low take-up in northern England and Scotland might be the result of a stronger culture of municipal welfare in traditional

Labour areas (McCurry, 1999). One commentator even suggested that such ideological concerns had created something of a 'north–south divide' (Pearson, 2000, p 463), with some northern English and Scottish authorities perceiving direct payments as a means of eroding public sector service provision, and Conservative-led authorities in southern England promoting direct payments as a means of encouraging individual choice and cost-efficiency (see Chapter Eight for further discussion).

The progression of implementation

Those new to direct payments might be surprised by how difficult it is to get access to meaningful data in this area. The way that different surveys have collected information has changed over time, making comparisons difficult – and compiling overall summaries of the experience across the UK can sometimes require going back to the original statistical sources (which are different – and not always easily accessible – in each country). The Direct Payments Survey in 2004 was the first UK-wide research on the implementation of direct payments, which comprised a postal questionnaire sent to all local authorities in the UK and another sent to 234 support organisations to gather information on all aspects of direct payments implementation and arrangements for support (Davey et al, 2007a–b). The survey was a collaborative project that combined the work of three separate research teams who were all involved in national studies of direct payments:

- *Disabled people and direct payments: a UK comparative study* (Riddell et al, 2006; see also Priestley et al, 2007);
- *An evaluation of the impact of the Social Care Modernisation Programme on the implementation of direct payments* [in England] (part of the DH Modernising Adult Social Care research initiative (MASC) (Vick et al, 2006);
- *Evaluation of the Direct Payments Development Fund implementation* funded by the Department of Health (Davey et al, 2007a–b).

These important research reports, published approximately a decade after the introduction of direct payments, showed a slow but steady increase in the overall take-up of direct payments and identified a number of ongoing issues:

- Despite having the lowest proportion of people in the UK with long-term illness or disability, England had established a more rapid take-up rate of direct payments than other parts of the UK (Riddell et al, 2006).
- The same study showed a similar regional pattern of direct payments in England as described earlier, with nine of the ten local authorities with the highest numbers of direct payments recipients located in the south or east of England (Riddell et al, 2005, p 80). The study concluded that direct payments were most strongly supported by central government within England and promoted there by Conservative-led local authorities. There had been scepticism in other

parts of the UK by local politicians and trade unions about direct payments aiding the privatisation of social care.

- Local cultures of welfare are important factors influencing local implementation, including the flexibility or otherwise of existing purchasing arrangements and the ease with which they can be changed (Riddell et al, 2006).

- Direct payment take-up figures showed a significant increase during the period that direct payments became mandatory in 2003/04. This statutory requirement was perceived as positive by local authorities but there was evidence of tension between the policy of increasing the take-up of direct payments and other policy initiatives (for example, to ration access to care; Vick et al, 2006).

- The change in regulations about the employment of close relatives in 2003 (see Chapter Three) was generally regarded as positive, particularly for those user groups who might find it difficult to access other assistance (Vick et al, 2006). However, there were also concerns about a range of difficulties that might arise through the payment of informal carers.

- Effective support schemes to assist people in setting up direct payments are critical. The DPDF (see Chapter Three) was seen as an important initiative, particularly in helping to target specific groups of service users. In the early days of implementation there was a strong correlation between those areas with a high take-up of direct payments and active user-led advocacy and support schemes but Riddell et al's (2006) study identified some concerns about the move of some user-led organisations away from advocacy and campaigning and towards direct service provision.

The current picture

More recent figures on the rate of take-up of direct payments show similar patterns to those described above. Tables 4.1–4.4 show a steady increase in the take up of direct payments in all four countries of the UK. The Association of Directors of Adult Social Services (ADASS) Personalisation Survey 2014 (completed by 132 or 87% of councils in England) estimates that 24% of people eligible to receive community-based services, and in receipt of a personal budget, now do so via a direct payment. Of the total budget spent by councils on personal budgets, 29% is spent on direct payments (ADASS, 2014, pp 10 and 14). As in the early years of implementation, regional variations are evident, with 21% of people receiving direct payments in the north east compared to 30% in the east Midlands (ADASS, 2014, p12).

A review by Hasler and Marshall (2013) of available research on the take-up of direct payments summarised the key factors that help promote payments (see Box 4.1; see also Chapters Seven and Eight). Their findings are not dissimilar to those identified in the first decade of the implementation of direct payments (see, for example, CSCI, 2004; Davey et al, 2007b), with good information and effective support schemes for potential recipients and training and support for front-line practitioners being crucial.

Table 4.1: Estimated number of adults in receipt of direct payments in England during the financial years 2008/09 to 2013/14*

Year	Number	Increase on previous year (%)
2008/09	86,000	n/a
2009/10*	107,000	25
2010/11	125,000	17
2011/12	139,000	11
2012/13	148,000	6
2013/14	155,000	5

* Figures for 2009/10 record the number of direct payments at only one point in the year, not over the whole financial year.

Source: Adapted from HSCIC, 2014, p 46, Figure 4.3.

Table 4.2: Estimated number of people in receipt of direct payments in Scotland during the financial years 2009/10 to 2013/14

Year	Number	Increase on previous year (%)
2009/10	3,678	n/a
2010/11	4,392	19
2011/12	5,049	15
2012/13	5,403	4
2013/14	6,010	11

Source: Adapted from Scottish Government, 2011 and 2014b.

Table 4.3: Estimated number of adults in receipt of direct payments in Wales during the financial years 2008/09 to 2013/14

Year	Number	Increase on previous year (%)
2008/09	2,265	n/a
2009/10	2,765	22
2010/11	3,085	48
2011/12	3,636	15
2012/13	4,134	14
2013/14	4,756	15

Source: Adapted from StatsWales, available online via https://statswales.wales.gov.uk/Catalogue/Health-and-Social-Care/Social-Services/Adult-Services/Service-Provision/AdultsReceivingServices-by-LocalAuthority-ClientCategory-Age (accessed 9 July 2015)

Table 4.4: Estimated number of people in receipt of direct payments in Northern Ireland in 2010–15*

Year	Number	Increase on previous year (%)
2010	1,864	n/a
2011	2,098	13
2012	2,423	15
2013	2,597	7
2014	2,770	7
2015	2,962	7

* Figures based on direct payments paid January–March each year including one-off paid and payments which ceased during the quarter.

Source: Adapted from CC8 Community Information return, DHSSPS, available online via http://www.dhsspsni.gov.uk/index/statistics/socialcare/direct-payments.htm (accessed 9 July 2015)

Box 4.1: Factors associated with increased take-up of direct payments

- Effective direct payments support schemes.
- Access to peer support to help build confidence and capacity.
- Advocacy for potential direct payment users.
- Making sure people are fully involved in the support planning process.
- Training and support for care managers and front-line staff.
- Leadership within local authorities.
- Accessible information on direct payments for service users and carers.
- Making sure people are kept informed about how their payments are managed and how much their budget is.
- Improving the information provided by councils about entitlements to social care services.
- Linking direct payments to overall commissioning strategies for personalisation.
- Ensuring that overall commissioning strategies reflect the qualities that people value in respect of services bought with direct payments.
- Ensuring applicants and recipients of direct payments receive earlier and better advocacy and independent support services.
- Streamlining local bureaucracy and offering access to support with administration of direct payments.
- Increased offering of family-led Independent Living Trusts, and other models for third party schemes.

(Hasler and Marshall, 2013, p 5)

The experience of different user groups

From the beginning, the strongest calls for reform came from people with physical impairments, and there is ongoing evidence to suggest that this group makes up the bulk of direct payments recipients. According to the Direct Payments Survey (Davey et al, 2007b, p 15):

- People with physical or sensory impairments were more likely to receive direct payments than any other service user group.
- The top five regions providing direct payments to this group had all had experience of early forms of indirect payments.
- The regional pattern of take-up by older people mirrored that of people with a physical or sensory impairment, albeit on a smaller scale.
- There were more people with learning difficulties receiving direct payments in the north-west of England than elsewhere, but the promotion of direct payments to this user group may have slowed as the focus turned to other groups.
- People with mental health problems were less likely to receive direct payments than any other group.

More recent figures for Scotland, Wales and Northern Ireland show a similar picture (see Tables 4.5–4.7), while the ADASS (2014) survey suggests that a much higher proportion of working-age disabled people receive a direct payment than do older people. Against this background, this chapter now looks briefly at the experiences of various user groups, considering some of the issues that have contributed to this uneven pattern of take-up. As indicated at the beginning of this chapter, there has been little research exclusively on direct payments since the second edition of this book. This section therefore summarises briefly the research findings that are still relevant as councils try to ensure greater equity between different user groups.

People with physical impairments

In many ways, the predominance of people with physical impairments receiving direct payments is unsurprising, since they have traditionally formed user groups that have been more powerful and politically active than those of other service users (M. Barnes, 1997). As a result, it was often people with physical impairments who were at the forefront of the campaign for direct payments, with early research suggesting that staff working with people with physical impairments were much more familiar with the concepts of independent living and direct payments than their colleagues in other settings (see, for example, Dawson, 2000). Indeed, the MASC study (Vick et al, 2006, p 70) found little evidence of champions of direct payments for any user groups *other* than people with physical impairments.

Table 4.5: Breakdown of adults in receipt of direct payments in Scotland during the financial year 2013/14

Service user group	Number – all ages	(%)
Physical disability	2,010	37
Learning disability	1,240	23
Frail older	1,110	21
Dementia	340	6
Mental health	290	5
Other	150	3
Physical disability and learning disability	140	3
N/K	100	2
TOTAL	5,390*	100

* Figures may not add up because of rounding.

Source: Adapted from Scottish Government, 2014b, pp 13 and 18.

Table 4.6: Breakdown of adults in receipt of direct payments in Wales during the financial year 2013/14

Service user group	Number – all ages	(%)
Physical disability	2,949	63
Learning disability	1,324	28
Mental health	319	7
Substance misuse	12	3
Other vulnerable groups	7	1
TOTAL	4,756	100*

* Figures may not add up because of rounding
Source: Adapted from StatsWales available online via https://statswales.wales.gov.uk/Catalogue/Health-and-Social-Care/Social-Services/Adult-Services/Service-Provision/AdultsReceivingServices-by-LocalAuthority-ClientCategory-Age (accessed 9 July 2015)

Table 4.7: Breakdown of adults in receipt of direct payments in Northern Ireland, 31 March 2015

Service user group	Number – all ages	(%)
Learning disability	948	32
Physical disability	902	30
Elderly care	843	28
Mental health	122	4
Carers	147	5
TOTAL	2,962	100*

* Figures may not add up because of rounding
Source: Adapted from CC8 Community Information return, DHSSPS available online via http://www.dhsspsni.gov.uk/index/statistics/socialcare/direct-payments.htm

Throughout the literature, it is the choice and control that direct payments enable that people with physical impairments seem to value the most (see, for example, the personal testimonies cited by Leece and Bornat, 2006). Service users interviewed by Shaping Our Lives, a national user-controlled organisation, said of direct payments:

> "It's given me my life back. Now I control who's helping me and when they come in. It's also given me a social life and I can do things I want to do."
>
> "When you employ your own personal assistants, you have more say and know what you're going to get, when." (Beresford et al, 2005, pp 24–5)

However, this does not change the fact that the number of direct payment recipients remains low compared to the number of people eligible, even among younger adults, who are most likely to receive a direct payment. In England on 31 March 2014, only 27% of people aged 18 to 64 eligible for community-based services had a direct payment (HSCIS, 2014, p 47).

Although the Carers and Disabled Children Act 2000 extended direct payments to 16- and 17-year-old disabled young people, exact figures about how many young people receive direct payments are hard to find and young disabled people have received little attention in the literature. Studies in 2003 by Scope, which included five young disabled adults (McMullen, 2003), and by JRF (Abbott, 2003), found that the majority of young disabled people identified independence as the key reason for applying for direct payments. They also identified a number of obstacles, including practical difficulties in accessing and managing direct payments and concerns from parents and professionals about whether young people would be able to manage their direct payments and how it would affect their relationship with their families (Abbott, 2003). More recently, a study conducted by SPRU, which interviewed 23 disabled young adults (Mitchell et al, 2015), many of whom received direct payments, reported similar findings, including the importance of social media in accessing peer support:

> So it was mainly personal networks that helped me, you know, understand what was going on ... I'm lucky to be able to speak with them on social media and talk it through. (Mitchell et al, 2015, p 2)

Nevertheless, for some disabled people, access remains difficult (Glynn et al, 2008). As an example, a key group whose needs are often overlooked are disabled parents, who may require additional hours as part of a direct payments care package for the physical aspects of parenting. A Social Care Institute for Excellence (SCIE) study (Morris and Wates, 2006) identified a lack of focus on the experiences of disabled adults as *parents* rather than as people using services, but highlighted the potential for direct payments to meet support needs better. The study found that funding for direct payments could also be difficult, sometimes falling between the remit of children's services and adult services (see also Morris and Wates, 2007).

People with learning difficulties

When direct payments legislation was being debated, the government's initial intention was to exclude people with learning difficulties until the new scheme could be tested in practice (DH/Scottish Office, Welsh Office/Northern Ireland Office, 1996; see Chapter Three). This restriction was eventually overturned following concerted lobbying by organisations such as People First, and subsequent guidance emphasised that local authorities should avoid blanket assumptions that whole groups of people are unable to manage payments (DH, 1997, 2000, 2003a). In practice, however, the number of people with learning difficulties receiving direct payments was initially small, with many people denied access (Fruin, 1998, 2000; Gardner, 1999) and a widespread assumption that direct payments would not work for people with learning difficulties (Dawson, 2000). Information about direct payments was also often unavailable in accessible formats and members of staff working with people with learning difficulties were frequently unaware of this way of working (Holman and Bewley, 1999; Maglajlic et al, 2000). Over time, the government has recognised the need for more accessible information and, as a result, produced extensive information both for local authorities and for people with learning difficulties to explain the concept of direct payments (see, for example, DH, 2004a–b, 2007).

Meanwhile, the number of people with learning difficulties receiving direct payments has been rising slowly; in England and Scotland the number of people with learning disabilities aged 18–64 is nearing the number of physically disabled people receiving a direct payment (HSCIC, 2014, p 56; Scottish Government, 2014b, p 18). The economic case for direct payments is compelling – the Direct Payments Survey found that, despite the average hourly rate for PAs for people with learning difficulties being higher than for other user groups, the average weekly live-in rates for people with learning difficulties were considerably lower than for weekly costs of residential care (Davey et al, 2007b, pp 58–61).

Even so, despite active encouragement by the government, the evidence suggests that people with learning difficulties continue to face a number of barriers. In the early days of direct payments, a recurring theme was the issue of consent, with many local authorities concerned and/or confused about the extent to which people with learning difficulties are able to consent to and manage direct payments (see Bewley, 1998; Ryan and Holman, 1998a–c; Holman and Bewley, 1999; Williams and Holman, 2006 for a more detailed discussion). In Scotland, this issue was overcome to a certain extent by the 2003 regulations extending direct payments to attorneys and guardians for people unable to manage their own payments (SSI 2003/243). In England, the Health and Social Care Act 2008 offered the opportunity to appoint a 'suitable person' to act on behalf of someone defined as lacking capacity (see Chapter Three), which may in part account for the increase in the number of people with learning disabilities receiving direct payments.

In addition to assistance in managing money, many people with learning difficulties (like all direct payment recipients) also need ongoing support. Peer support in particular can be very effective in inspiring other people with learning difficulties to see the potential opportunities that direct payments can bring (Bewley and McCulloch, 2004). However, evidence to date suggests that many support schemes focus more on the take-up and setting up of direct payments, rather than on maintenance and ongoing management (which are often left to the recipient themselves – see Davey et al, 2007a).

Mental health

The initial neglect of mental health issues was apparent from the early stages of the implementation of direct payments – indeed, as the Direct Payments Bill was being debated in Parliament, there were specific (unsuccessful) attempts to *exclude* all service users with mental health problems (Beresford, 1996). While these were defeated, it is perhaps unsurprising that subsequent numbers remained low (Maglajlic, 1999; Witcher et al, 2000; Heslop, 2001). Key barriers have been found to include lack of knowledge among service users, staff and carers, high eligibility criteria for receiving any support and difficulties managing money when ill (Maglajlic et al, 1998; Maglajlic, 1999). Research commissioned by the Scottish Executive echoed many of these findings but particularly highlighted unfavourable staff attitudes and misunderstandings about eligibility for direct payments as 'formidable barrier[s] to access for mental health service users' (Ridley and Jones, 2003, p 650).

The Department of Health (DH) admitted that the situation in 2005 was unacceptable as almost a quarter of local authorities in England were making no direct payments to people with mental health problems, and a further half were making between one and five. According to the National Institute for Mental Health in England (NIMHE) (2006, p 3): '*it is time for action*' (emphasis in the original). The government therefore commissioned new guidance for a range of key stakeholders (NIMHE, 2006) and funded projects in five local authorities to promote independent living via direct payments for people with mental health problems (Spandler and Vick, 2006; see also Davidson and Luckhurst, 2002). At the start of the project there were no mental health service users in the pilot sites and by the end there were 58. In the evaluation the recipients reported significant benefits that direct payments offered in relation to increased opportunities and greater independence. However, despite this, 'only a very small number of mental health professionals had really grasped the principles of direct payments and independent living and were generally promoting it as a positive option to service users' (Spandler and Vick, 2006, p 112). Professionals were selective both in whom they offered direct payments to and also in what they agreed they should be used for.

Based on this work, the Health and Social Care Advisory Service undertook a project, 'New Directions', to promote the use of direct payments by people with mental health problems, including those from black and minority ethnic communities (Newbigging with Lowe, 2005). The project brought together service users, practitioners, senior managers and voluntary organisations with service users recruited to facilitate the groups. The practical and organisational barriers identified by the participants confirmed those outlined above, but the study highlighted additional obstacles faced by mental health service users from black and minority ethnic groups. These included language and cultural issues, inconsistency and inequality in the practices of different local authorities, and evidence that participants felt reflected 'institutional racism and notions about mental ill health and black people' (Newbigging with Lowe, 2005, p 19).

In addition to general barriers for all users, the Direct Payments Survey identified a number of specific issues for mental health service users:

- Particular difficulties were reported over the episodic nature of some people's mental ill health, and it may not always be appropriate to offer direct payments when people are in crisis (Vick et al, 2006, p 56). In this and other studies there was little evidence of advance directives being used to indicate what people wanted to happen at a time of crisis (Spandler and Vick, 2006).
- Lack of resources can limit how people go about meeting needs. Indeed, the Direct Payments Survey found that, generally, care packages were smaller for mental health service users than for other service user groups, with fewer than half of mental health users getting more than ten hours per week (Davey et al, 2007b, p 45). However, for some people such a short time *can* make a difference: 'I used to attend a day centre five days a week, but this was not stimulating and my five hours now are more valuable than five days used to be' (Newbigging with Lowe, 2005, p 23).
- There were difficulties meeting needs that fell between the boundaries of both health and social care and with agreeing financial responsibilities (Vick et al, 2006, p 69; see also Taylor, 2008).
- Appropriate support from people who had detailed knowledge, understanding and expertise in mental health issues was not readily available to recipients in either setting up or managing direct payments (Vick et al, 2006, p 66; see also Newbigging with Lowe, 2005).

However, the concerns of some professionals expressed in the research above are in stark contrast to accounts by service users of the ability of direct payments to transform the lives of people who have previously been disempowered and who have not been able to obtain a satisfactory response to their needs from directly provided statutory services (Davidson and Luckhurst, 2002; Newbigging with Lowe, 2005; Spandler and Vick, 2006).

Older people

When direct payments were first implemented, they were initially prohibited for people aged 65 or over (unless the person had been receiving payments before the age of 65). Sustained pressure from disabled people's and older people's organisations about the discriminatory nature of this approach (NCIL, ndb, 1999; Age Concern, 1998) encouraged New Labour to extend direct payments to people aged 65 and over (DH, 1998b; see also Chapter Three), a decision also welcomed by the Royal Commission on Long-Term Care (1999).

Since then, the take-up of direct payments by older people has been relatively low (Riddell et al, 2006). In England, in 2013/14 approximately 63,000 older received direct payments (HSCIC, 2014, p 34) with striking regional variations. A report commissioned by Think Local Act Personal (TLAP – a national partnership of health and social care organisations committed to transforming health and care through personalisation and community-based support) reports: '12 councils have direct payment levels over 20% for over 65s but 16 councils are achieving under 4%' (Routledge et al, 2015, p 6). The ADASS 2014 survey highlights that although older people are the biggest group of people who have been allocated personal budgets (51%), only 15% of them have direct payments, as compared to 37% of younger adults. From the beginning, early experience suggested that older people could be put off direct payments by some of the difficulties (both real and perceived) of administering them, in particular the responsibilities of becoming an employer (Zarb and Oliver, 1993; C. Barnes, 1997; Hasler et al, 1999). In 2004, a key study that explored how direct payments were operating for older people was undertaken by Clark et al (2004) in three local authorities. Typically at that time, providing direct payments was not part of care managers' usual way of working. While some were enthusiastic about the prospect, others identified major difficulties that related to the workload and tight eligibility criteria, but primarily the 'nature of the client group' – with many older people felt by workers to be too frail to manage direct payments (Clark et al, 2004, p 40). Some of the main findings are listed below:

- The majority of people chose direct payments in preference to directly provided services in order to have more choice and control over support arrangements or because it was the only way they could get what they needed.
- All the older people reported positive outcomes for their physical health or sense of well-being.
- Having someone speak their own language and understand their cultural needs was important for older people from minority ethnic communities.
- Handling the relationship with their PA was the key to managing direct payments well, and having access to an effective support scheme was crucial.

These issues are similar to those from other studies (for example, Glendinning et al, 2000a; CSCI, 2004; Poole, 2006; Vick et al, 2006). A more recent study published by TLAP (Routledge and Carr, 2013) to explore the challenges and to identify good practice in improving personal budgets for older people found some familiar reasons why older people and carers were reluctant to take up direct payments, including:

- satisfaction with existing services;
- reluctance to take on 'management', including employees;
- complexity of rules and arrangements;
- time-consuming processes;
- concern about possible reduction of services.

The report identifies where councils are reviewing and adapting their current policies and processes in relation to direct payments in order to make them more attractive to older people. These include: the introduction of pre-payment cards to avoid the person having to administer a separate bank account; clear and more accurate advice and information given at the right time; and development of more effective peer support schemes (for a full account of the challenges and local responses see Routledge and Carr, 2013 and a follow-up TLAP report by Routledge et al, 2015). Both these sources also identify critical workforce issues which may determine whether or not older people are enabled to consider direct payments. Issues include staff not thinking direct payments are appropriate for older people, feeling under-skilled, or not being used to establishing long-term relationships with older people. An additional issue is around timing (Scourfield, 2005b; Age UK, 2010), with many older people meeting professionals for the first time when they are in crisis (which may be a bad time for an in-depth conversation about options such as direct payments). This raises a crucial dilemma about when and how best to have such conversations, with the danger that direct payments are not mentioned on first contact with services and then are not mentioned again (see Chapter Eight for further discussion of the gatekeeping role of social workers).

People with dementia

The Health and Social Care Act 2008 has made it possible for people with dementia who lack capacity to receive direct payments via the appointment of a 'suitable person' (see Chapter Three). Before then the Direct Payments Survey estimated that 0.1% of older people receiving direct payments had mild to moderate dementia (Davey et al, 2007b, p 36). Subsequent accurate data is hard to find. The most extensive study was undertaken in 2010 by the Alzheimer's Society, which surveyed 1,432 people with dementia and their carers in England, Wales and Northern Ireland. A total of 878 people were receiving social care services, and of those 204 (23%) said they were in receipt of personal budgets or direct payments (Lakey and Saunders, 2011). A small study of 12 carers of direct payment recipients estimates there may be approximately 300 direct payments made for people with dementia in Scotland (Kinnaird and Fearnley, 2010).

The Alzheimer's Society study found that people with dementia who were living with carers were more likely to be receiving direct payments than older people living alone, as were younger people with dementia and their carers. Payments were most often used for employing care staff at home, helping with personal care and offering respite services (Lakey and Saunders, 2011). Overall (pp iii–iv):

- Respondents who accessed direct payments were more likely to be satisfied with services than those who did not. This related to being able to recruit and train their own carers and having flexibility in what the carers could do that better suited the person's needs
- Accessing and using direct payments presented many challenges, including overly complex administration, lack of knowledge among key staff (particularly in relation to people with dementia who lack capacity) and eligibility criteria that meant that services were sometimes available only at the point of crisis.
- More people with dementia could benefit from direct payments, but only if timely and appropriate support is in place.
- Direct payments are not suitable for all and there must be other ways that people with dementia and their carers can still have some choice and control over services.

Similar findings were reported by Laybourne et al (2014), who undertook a small study of seven 'suitable people' who were managing a direct payment for someone who could not consent and nine social care practitioners. Because of their focus on the role of the suitable people they made other reflections which, despite the exploratory nature of the study, make an important contribution to this little-researched area:

- While practitioners could see the flexibility that direct payments brought to people with dementia, there was concern about the attitudes of some workers, typified by the comment, 'everybody, every member of staff, all the different disciplines, don't really think it's for our clientele' (p 8).
- Suitable people were not always clear about the assessment processes that were being used and were not confident that the views of the person with dementia had been represented, particularly if they (the suitable person) had not been present to help interpret their responses.
- Services bought by direct payments often benefitted people with dementia *and* their carers. Where these two interests converged this was not problematic, but where their interests were in conflict, the person with dementia had to remain the focus for the suitable person. This may in some cases preclude the carer from acting as the suitable person.

The limited research in this area suggests that direct payments can be of benefit to people with dementia in the same ways as for many other people. However, standard assessment and support-planning processes may not be suitable for people with dementia and there may be useful lessons to be learnt from work with people with learning disabilities about the use of person–centred planning techniques (Laybourne et al, 2014, p 14).

Carers

Following changes in legislation in 2001, carers aged over 16 are eligible to receive direct payments in their own right. In 2013/14, 47,000 carers in England receiving services through a self-directed support process did so through a direct payment, an impressive increase of 46% from the previous year (HSCIS, 2014, p 58). However, these figures should be treated with caution as there may be some confusion about the classification of direct payments in some areas – for example, the MASC study reported: 'In one apparently high performing authority, over 90% of payments to people with mental health needs were actually one-off payments to provide respite for carers. Hence the figures for service users can appear inflated whilst carer figures are undercounted' (Vick et al, 2006, p 37). The same study also found that, while direct payments were small in numbers, there were a high proportion of one-off payments to carers which are not always apparent in the figures (Vick et al, 2006). Box 4.2 gives an example of how one-off payments have helped to support carers.

Box 4.2: Flexible use of a carer's one-off direct payment

Connor has been caring for his wife, who is in a wheelchair with ME and arthritis, for the last nine years. He does all the cooking, driving and general household duties for her. Connor received a personal budget which he requested in the form of a direct payment from his local authority for a laptop to enable him to be in more regular contact through Skype with family in the US. This now enables Connor to stay connected with family he cannot afford to fly and see. This family support helps Connor with his ongoing caring role.

Divya has four young children and provides care for her father who is nearing the end of his life. Her father receives a direct payment, which he used to pay for a family member to come from India for a period of time to give his daughter a break from her caring role. Divya received a carer's direct payment, which she uses for her children to attend summer play schemes so that she can get some free time to meet with friends and socialise when the Indian family member provides care to her father. This gives Divya regular breaks from caring which are important to the family unit.

(DH, 2014a, p 160)

A recent small study on the impact of personal budgets, including direct payments, on carers of older people and people with learning disabilities reported that carers, while involved in the assessment and support of people for whom they cared, much less frequently had their own needs assessed and met, particularly in relation to leisure, training and employment (Glendinning et al, 2015). These findings are similar to earlier evidence that 'overall, the emphasis is on using direct payments to support carers to continue caring, rather than to support their fulfilment as citizens' (CSCI, 2008a, p 100).

For some, the opportunity to employ family members has proved useful. While there are mixed views about this (see Chapter Eight), many carers would echo the words of this woman:

> "My husband will not be looked after by anyone he doesn't know … Hence I have really never had a break … My daughter can be the carer so that is good as she knows my husband's illness so well." (Fletcher, 2006, p 182)

Despite this, a scoping review of literature in 2010 found: 'there is surprisingly little information on the management and negotiations of employment relationships, particularly when family members step into paid roles' (Manthorpe et al, 2011a, p 204). While much of the evidence suggests that direct payments can contribute to good outcomes for carers, therefore, the eight lessons for local authorities identified by Carers UK in 2008 are still relevant (p 10):

1. Speed up the application process.
2. Make it a real choice. Direct payments are not right for every care situation and no one should feel pressured into accepting them.
3. Provide employment support.
4. Make sure all costs are covered.
5. Allow families to employ family members.
6. Don't back off, back up [with] appropriate back up and contingency plans in place before a carer is required to manage the direct payment independently.
7. Value carers' administrative support.
8. Keep commissioning highly specialist services.

Parents of disabled children

When direct payments were extended to the parents of disabled children, the issue had received little attention from local authority children's services. Christine Lenehan, director of the Council for Disabled Children, believed this was because direct payments 'were an adult-based concept plonked on children, and it took quite a while to untangle what they meant for children' (quoted in Vevers, 2007).

To date, particular barriers in children's services appear to include the relatively underdeveloped nature of the 'market', with seemingly fewer alternatives to directly provided services. There is also some evidence to suggest that demand for assessments has increased as a result of direct payments, although it is not clear whether this is because of the reduced stigma attached to direct payments, dissatisfaction with current services or an expectation that direct payments will meet needs more appropriately (Carlin and Lenehan, 2004). However, Welch et al (2011) surveyed 348 parents and carers with children using short breaks (of whom 90 were using direct payments) and found the use of direct payments was 'inequitably distributed with higher level of use by families in less deprived areas, carers with higher levels of education, White British carers, female carers and families with younger children' (Welch et al, 2011 p 907; see also Chapter Eight for discussion on inequity). Despite this, those parents who have successfully accessed direct payments often seem to have benefitted. In one study in the north-west, key positives included:

- *Flexibility*: "I can use support money in different ways. I can find different styles of care ... I am able to select the carer and the types of care."
- *Appropriate type of care*: for example, recruiting a carer of the same sex to pursue the child's interest in football.
- *Effective use of a small amount of money*: over three-quarters of the sample were receiving only between £20 and £50, but had been able to utilise it in innovative ways that had both given the family a break and given the child a chance to get involved in local community activities.
- *Less involvement with a range of professionals*: one respondent commented, "I don't want a social worker; I just need some money to help us have an ordinary family life" (Blyth and Gardner, 2007, pp 238–9).

Similarly, a father interviewed for a SCIE knowledge review of the social care needs of children with complex health care needs and their families said:

> "The direct payment scheme has really transformed our family. Previously it was a struggle getting the help we needed but since direct payments we have been able to employ people who are fit, warm-natured, happy to be trained by us and willing to work with our schedules, for example, starting late on some mornings or accompanying us on holidays." (Marchant et al, 2007, p 22)

Overall, Blyth and Gardner (2007) identify five key messages for local authorities that are seeking to increase the take-up of direct payments by parents of disabled children:

- Arrange for independently managed direct payment support services to help with practical and emotional support.
- Direct payments need 'champions' – a senior manager who will develop a clear authority-wide strategy and drive it forward, and also at practitioner level to inspire confidence in other staff.

- Recruit 'recipient champions' who can promote direct payments and help share their experiences with others.
- Recipients in this study found the ability to employ close relatives very positive, and an empowering experience for parents of disabled children to be managing rather than receiving services.
- Setting up an effective direct payments scheme needs *additional* resources in order to cope with a potential increase in demand for services, set up a suitable support scheme and train staff appropriately. Only then can a sustainable scheme be established.

However, a hint of warning still remains from Carlin and Lenehan's study: 'direct payments represent a significant change to the philosophy or underlying ethos of children's services. This barrier is key and councils are going to need significant reassurance that they can really let go and trust parents with direct payments' (2006, p 121).

Seldom-heard groups

In addition to the main groups above, direct payments hold out the potential to reach a range of people excluded from or treated less favourably by directly provided services. While these are often described as 'hard to reach', we prefer the term 'seldom heard' as it seems to us to reflect more accurately the difficulty the system sometimes has in engaging with and responding to the needs of these groups. By definition, the following overview is very brief, but it seems at least possible that direct payments could have a potential impact on five particular groups:

- *People with complex and fluctuating needs*: Henwood and Hudson (2009) identify the potential benefits and challenges of direct payments for people with complex and multiple needs. Taking a longitudinal approach (rather than a one-off review at a particular moment in time), Arksey and Baxter (2012) worked with 30 direct payment recipients over the course of two years, including young people with life-limiting conditions, working-age people and older people with fluctuating conditions. This study identified that people needed: opportunities to talk about longer-term issues of care from the start of the process; ongoing support with managing direct payments, including the flexibility to manage the money as their needs fluctuated; knowledgeable practitioners to give advice and information but also support from 'expert direct payments recipients' (Arksey and Baxter, 2012, p 162).
- *People with HIV/AIDS*: while there is little data on the number and experience of people with HIV/AIDS receiving direct payments, preliminary work undertaken by NCIL and the National AIDS Trust suggested that direct payments may be a particularly positive option, leading to greater flexibility, improved continuity, more control and improved health as fluctuating needs

are met more effectively (Grimshaw and Fletcher, nd). One social work team in the MASC study reported that direct payments were particularly useful for black African service users with HIV (Vick et al, 2006, p 64). What was important here was the flexibility and choice for the individual to employ someone of their choosing. For some, this was a trusted friend or relative, while others preferred someone outside their immediate community as a result of concerns about privacy and confidentiality.

- *Lesbian, gay, bisexual and trans-gender people (LGBT)*: in an early paper on 'Independent living, personal assistance, disabled lesbians and disabled gay men', Killin (1993) sets out some of the practical issues faced by gay and lesbian PA users, including discriminatory attitudes by PAs and the difficulty of knowing when to disclose their sexuality to their PA. Many of these issues were subsequently reiterated in PSI/NCIL guidance to local authorities (Hasler et al, 1999, pp 32–3), emphasising the need to consider the importance of peer support, maintaining confidentiality and specific measures to consult disabled lesbians and gay men seeking to live independently. A report by CSCI in 2008 on the needs of LGBT people using social care services found direct payments were popular in order to help ensure positive attitudes through choice of worker; flexibility over times to engage in social events; and control in deciding what to do if a worker acts in a discriminatory manner (CSCI, 2008b). Although they faced a number of challenges, LGBT people receiving direct payments expressed a higher level of satisfaction than did people receiving traditional services.

- *People living in rural areas*: opinion is currently divided on the implications of direct payments for people in rural areas. While some believe that the flexibility of direct payments may be a positive way of trying to meet needs in places poorly served by directly provided services, others point to the complexities of recruiting staff and the cost of travelling to and from people's homes. However, it does appear as though the relaxation of rules on employing close relatives has been helpful for older people in rural areas who may want to employ family members living near to them (Vick et al, 2006, p 37; Larsen et al, 2013, p 179). Similar findings were reported by a Commission for Rural Communities study (2008) into the implications of personalisation for rural older people, which also stresses the importance of contingency planning when arranging home-based services in rural areas – 'Plan B' must be ready to put into place if a PA is sick or unable to work. While the evidence is limited, our view is that many of the barriers cited in the literature apply equally to both direct payments and directly provided services, but that direct payments may provide additional flexibility when seeking ways of overcoming some of these issues.

- *Black and minority ethnic communities*: experience to date suggests that direct payments may be a good way of meeting the needs of people from minority ethnic groups and may compare favourably with direct services (Hasler et al, 1999; Clark et al, 2004; Stuart, 2006; Vick et al, 2006; Davey et al, 2007b). Despite this, there is also evidence to suggest that people from minority ethnic groups may face additional barriers to accessing direct payments and remain under-represented (Butt and Box, 1997; Bignall and Butt, 2000; Butt et al, 2000; Maglajlic et al, 2000; Witcher et al, 2000; Stuart, 2006). In particular, research by SCIE (Stuart, 2006, p ix) identifies a range of issues, including:

- assessment processes not taking account of black and minority ethnic service users' backgrounds and requirements;
- service users being unaware of how to access or use information on direct payments;
- difficulty in recruiting PAs;
- shortage of appropriate advocacy and support services;
- variable levels of commitment to direct payments among local authorities.

Within the broader literature there is much debate about the role of the family, and in particular the relaxation of the rule on employing close relatives. Some people argue that black and Asian people may wish to employ family members as PAs in order to obtain a more culturally sensitive service, while others feel that this would blur the role of family members and reduce the independence of the disabled person. However, a finding that is consistent throughout the literature is the importance of providing appropriate and adequate support for people from minority ethnic groups to find out about, access and manage direct payments (see Vick et al, 2006 for some positive examples).

International experience

Although this book focuses on the UK, it is easy to lose sight of the fact that the move towards forms of more individualised funding is something of an international trend. Although the following account cannot provide a detailed summary, the remainder of this chapter offers a brief flavour of the experience in some other countries, citing further references for those interested in following up specific examples in more detail. Cash-for-care schemes (of which direct payments are one example) have become a key feature of European social policy (Da Roit and Le Bihan, 2010; Glendinning, 2010) and Table 4.8 shows the key features of some cash payment schemes across Europe and the US, illustrating the type of programme available, take-up and whether relatives may be employed (Poole, 2006, p 6).

In an analysis of schemes in six European countries, Da Roit and Le Bihan (2010, p 286) identified four common objectives for cash payment schemes:

- to promote choice of the type of care for the service user;
- to promote improved quality and efficiency in care provision because of increased competition;
- to give recognition and payment to informal carers (and in some countries family members);
- to contain costs of long-term care for disabled people.

Table 4.8: Take-up of individualised funding

Country	Type of programme	Employment of relatives?	Percentage of 65+ population in receipt of social care who have direct payments or a personal budget
Austria	Cash allowance	Yes	100*
Germany	Option of cash allowance or care-in-kind or a combination of the two	Yes	80 (including those who choose a care package that combines cash and services)
Luxembourg	Option of a cash allowance to cover first 7hrs/week of care	Yes	91 (including those who choose a care package that combines cash and services)
Sweden	Cash payment; minimum need of 17hrs/week	Yes	1
Netherlands	Personal budget – since April 2003 available to all those qualifying for long-term home-based care	Yes (but not in the same home)	7
Norway	Personal budget for care assistants when local authority considers this a better option than formal agency care	Yes	2
United States	Medicaid pay for a specified number of hours of a user-hired personal assistant	Yes (but not spouses)	18

Source: Poole, 2006, p 6 adapted from Lundsgaard, 2005.
* The Austrian system is closer to the UK equivalent of Attendance Allowance than direct payments/personal budgets.

There are, however, significant differences between countries, dependent upon the context in which they are introduced. In the Netherlands, personal budgets were piloted in 1995, partly as a response to pressure from service users for greater autonomy and flexibility, and became policy in 2001. As in France, the use of these payments is heavily regulated with restrictions on how they are used, including where family carers are employed. By contrast, in Germany, Italy and Austria, where the employment of close relatives is also allowed, but where more informal arrangements are acceptable, 'recipients are free to spend their benefits as they wish' (Da Roit and Le Bihan, 2010, p 299). Partly as a result of this, in these three countries an unregulated grey labour market of care workers has developed, largely staffed by immigrant female workers (Da Roit and Le Bihan, 2010; see also Chapter Eight for a discussion of gender). However, as Glendinning (2010, p 45) points out:

> Pressures on service providers may be reduced if cash allowances are used to support family care or (in the case of some countries) employ migrant 'grey' labour. Furthermore, the implications for informal carers may be less positive if the care they provide is regarded as a substitute for formal service provision.

While the form and scope of cash-for-care payments vary considerably, research commissioned by the European Association for Care and Help at Home has found that the same key questions have been asked in most countries:

- Will more people apply for cash than for services?
- Should allowances become part of a social insurance system or should it be social assistance?
- What is the best way to assess an applicant and to determine the amount to be paid?
- Will the recipients of cash use it properly?
- Will the quality of services bought with the cash be adequate?
- Will PAs be treated well by their employers? (Pijl, 2000, pp 56–7)

In the US and Canada the context of direct funding for people receiving social care services is rather different (see Lord and Hutchinson, 2003; Hutchinson et al, 2006). Direct payments had a much earlier inception than in Europe, and Hutchinson et al (2006, p 49) describe 'individualised planning and direct funding as [having] evolved as cornerstones of a new paradigm of disability supports for citizenship and inclusion'. Unlike in the UK, the movement in North America has been driven by piecemeal local initiatives (Hutchinson et al, 2006, p 52). In reviewing the lessons learnt from this experience, Hutchinson et al (2006, pp 56–60) identify a number of key factors:

- the importance of values and principles that reflect self-determination and community participation in driving any direct funding initiative;
- policy frameworks are key to guiding change but are currently limited in North America;
- the power of independent planning support to build and sustain capacity for self-funding initiatives;
- non-bureaucratic, simple funding approaches that ideally can move between areas are important;
- small-scale change informs system change – the challenge is how to reproduce and maintain the values and principles evident in small-scale projects in building a larger, more comprehensive service system that addresses individualised planning and direct funding.

Finally, SCIE (2007) has produced a research briefing that gives a helpful overview of the UK and international literature on consumer-directed payments. Key issues include:

- the different models of support that different countries have found most useful – for example, a review of ten initiatives in Canada, Australia and the US found that support systems independent from service delivery were most helpful;
- the huge increase in demand for PAs has been apparent in all countries;

- issues of low wages for PAs and an unregulated market are common throughout;
- almost all countries have underestimated the costs of schemes and many have had to contain the rising demand for cash payments.

However, the concluding observation of the review is that: 'Consumer satisfaction and reported growth in autonomy have been the most frequently reported outcomes of consumer–directed care' (p 9).

SUMMARY

Early on, the progress of direct payments was uneven, with more rapid implementation in the south of England than in the north, Wales, Northern Ireland and many parts of Scotland. Key barriers appear to have included fears about the erosion of public services, a lack of awareness among social workers, financial concerns and a lack of accessible information (among others). When direct payments became mandatory, the number of recipients increased and the pace of change quickened. However, direct payments have sometimes been conceptualised from the perspective of people with physical impairments, and people from other service user groups have sometimes been excluded from, or found it difficult to access, payment schemes. Although different groups face different obstacles, recurring themes include a lack of appropriate information and support, unsupportive professionals, bureaucratic procedures and concerns about becoming an employer. Despite these barriers, forms of individualised funding have also been introduced in a number of other countries, and the UK experience is by no means unique.

IMPLICATIONS FOR POLICY AND PRACTICE

- Direct payments have spread unevenly across different geographical areas and among different user groups. Often this seems to be to do with the way in which direct payments have been operationalised, and the history and culture of specific services.
- A key role is played by front-line workers, who act as gatekeepers to this system. This is explored in more detail in Chapter Eight, but the attitude and approach of individual practitioners may well be crucial to whether the option of direct payments is raised in a constructive way (or even raised at all).
- The role of support services is crucial (see also Chapter Eight) – the role of peer support, accessible information, ongoing support over time and positive role models can be particularly important.
- A senior 'champion' can be helpful in securing resources and maintaining profile. At the level of front-line practice, a practice 'champion' can inspire and encourage staff who may be uncertain or ambivalent about their role in helping people access direct payments.
- Although this chapter has tended to focus on overall numbers and trends, direct payments are only a means to an end; the quality of people's individual experience is more important than quantity per se.

RECOMMENDED READING AND USEFUL WEBSITES

For a national overview of the recent spread and impact of direct payments:

* ADASS conducts an annual survey that gives a national overview of the progress of personalisation in local authorities, including the number of people receiving direct payments (www.adass.org.uk/home).
* HSCIS produces an annual report of social care activity in local authorities, including the cost and take-up of direct payments – the Community Care Statistics, Social Services Activity, England (www.hscic.gov.uk).
* Hasler and Marshall (2013) provide an overview of recent research on direct payments with respect to the views of social care managers, service users and carers and the state of support services for recipients of direct payments.

For previous national overviews, see:

* Riddell et al's (2006) comparative study of direct payments in the four countries of the UK;
* Vick et al's (2006) national study on the implementation of direct payments;
* Davey et al's (2007a–b) national surveys of direct payments policy and practice.

For an overview of the experience of different user groups, see:

* Mitchell et al (2015) (for younger disabled people);
* Williams and Holman (2006) (for people with learning difficulties);
* Taylor (2008) (for people with mental health problems);
* Poldervaart and Malenczuk (2013) (for older people);
* Lakey and Saunders (2011) (for people with dementia)
* Carers UK (2008) (for carers);
* Carlin and Lenehan (2006) (for parents of disabled children);
* Stuart (2006) (for black and minority ethnic communities);
* Commission for Rural Communities (2008) (for rural communities).

For international lessons, see:

* Lundsgaard's (2005) OECD review;
* SCIE's (2007) review of the international literature on direct payments;
* Da Roit and Le Bihan's analysis of cash-for-care schemes in six European countries.

REFLECTIVE EXERCISES

1. Looking back, it is easy to be critical of the slow and uneven pace at which direct payments sometimes spread. However, how do you think you would have reacted at the time if you had been a worker trying to find out about direct payments and support service users to explore such a new way of working?

2. If you work or are on placement in a local authority, how easy is it for workers and for service users to find accessible information about direct payments? How easy is it to access peer support and to find positive role models?

3. Talk to people with experience of receiving direct payments – what has helped or hindered them?

4. Reflecting on the different user groups discussed in this chapter (including seldom heard groups), to what extent can direct payments help to overcome traditional barriers and improve access to support?

FIVE

Personal budgets – where they came from and why they matter

This chapter explores:
- the history and evolution of personal budgets;
- key features, concepts and values;
- emerging evidence about impact.

Although direct payments and personal budgets are often seen as two sides of the same coin, they are actually entirely separate ways of working (albeit with much in common). As explained in previous chapters, direct payments involve the payment of the cash equivalent of a directly provided service to a person eligible for social care, who then uses this to design their own support. They are the result of a longstanding campaign by disabled people and their organisations, and now have a long track record (with indirect payments in place for many years and direct payments formally in place since 1996). While personal budgets build on such history, they are more recent in their introduction (from 2003) and originated from allies of the disabled people's movement working within services for people with learning difficulties, rather than from disabled people themselves.

At its most simple, a personal budget involves being clear with the person at the start how much money is available to meet their needs, then allowing them maximum choice over how this money is spent on their behalf and over how much control they want over the money itself. While this could result in the person taking the full personal budget as a direct payment, there are several other ways of organising support (which can include a social worker managing the full amount on the person's behalf). Thus, the money need not actually change hands – the key is that the person knows immediately how much is likely to be spent on their needs, and can then be more creative in thinking of new ways to meet these needs. For all the debate that personal budgets have generated, this seems to us to be little more than 'sensible delegation' (personal communication, In Control) – ensuring that the person with the biggest vested interest in making a support package work as effectively as possible is able to control how that support is organised and delivered. Another key difference from direct payments is that personal budgets can be spent on anything that can be shown to be meeting a person's assessed needs – and this can include a combination of public, private and voluntary sector services (including things that do not look like traditional 'services' at all). Perhaps most importantly of all, direct payments sometimes felt like a very empowering way of working bolted on to traditional and unresponsive systems. While direct payments can transform the way in which people receive support, they have not changed the way in which people access services, the way they are assessed, the prevailing culture or the way in which the bulk of the social care budget is spent. In contrast, personal budgets, when they were first introduced, seemed to offer all the advantages of direct payments, while also holding out the potential for transforming the system as a whole. It is for a combination of these reasons – because they were so new, because they derived from different sources to direct payments, because they are easy to confuse with direct payments and because they aim at broader system change – that personal budgets have tended to attract strong responses – both positive and negative.

History and evolution

Although direct payments and personal budgets have a different history and focus, both have been greeted with high expectations by people using services and their allies. Following on from the high hopes that many people had for direct payments (see the quotation at the start of Chapter One from Oliver and Sapey, 1999), personal budgets and self-directed support have been described as 'potentially the biggest change to the provision of social care in England in 60 years' (Browning, 2007, p 3). Beginning initially within services for people with learning difficulties, the advent of personal budgets was closely linked to the aspirations of *Valuing People*, New Labour's strategy for learning disability services (DH, 2001f). Unlike many other policy documents, *Valuing People* did not focus on health and social care as an end in themselves, but on a broader vision for people's lives (with health and social care merely as a means to these ends). As set out in Box 5.1, the central focus was on four key principles: rights, choice, independence and inclusion. Given the history of social care summarised in Chapter Two, the commitment to such principles was always likely to lead to tension with the traditional social care system (which contained very few formal rights and relatively little choice, with rather a mixed track record with regard to independence and inclusion). While *Valuing People* brought a helpful focus to these debates, however, the history of personal budgets is inextricably linked with a group of people and calls for reform that might be described as an 'inclusion movement'. Although this approach receives much less attention than the more well-known concept of independent living, it draws many of its ideas from concepts such as supported living, person-centred planning and self-advocacy and sets the context within which *Valuing People*, personal budgets and self-directed support must be viewed.

Against this background, the concept of personal budgets was first developed by a small group of individuals meeting in 2003 to discuss ways of working within the current social care system to bring about the biggest possible change for people with learning difficulties. While this is described in more detail in Box 5.2, many of these early pioneers had a long track record of working to support people with learning difficulties to leave long-stay hospitals and live independently in the community. Throughout this previous work, a key frustration had been that the barrier to further progress always seemed to be the fact that so much of the money available was tied up in existing buildings and in pre-paid services, rather than available to use flexibly and creatively to support people in the community. In this way, what were later to become personal budgets began life as an attempt to think of radical new ways of doing things that would nevertheless be compatible with the current legal and financial framework.

Box 5.1: *Valuing People*

In 2001, *Valuing People* (DH, 2001f) set out a new vision for learning disability services in the twenty-first century. The first such policy document since 1971, *Valuing People* emphasised the importance of four key principles:

- rights
- choice
- independence
- control.

Individual chapters of the strategy then focused on topics such as disabled children and young people; choice and control; supporting carers; improving health; housing, fulfilling lives and employment; quality services; partnership working; and making change happen. In particular, *Valuing People* argued that current services are characterised by variable quality; shortfalls in provision of particular services; varying degrees of commitment by local authorities and the NHS; and widespread isolation and social exclusion. Instead, the strategy proposed a series of radical changes to a broad range of services designed to improve the lives of people with learning difficulties and their families; promote choice, social inclusion and independence; and recognise people's rights as citizens.

From these initial discussions came a new way of organising social care (self-directed support), based on a new way of allocating resources and on a new way of enabling the individual to be in control of their support. As Box 5.3 suggests, self-directed support is based on a series of seven steps. While the principles and concepts associated with personal budgets are explored in more detail below, the main point here is that the personal budget, so often the focus of discussion, is only part of a much broader attempt to transform the social care system as a whole – it is not an end in itself. Borrowing language and concepts from the manufacture of computer software, In Control described this as a new 'operating system' that is 'open-source' in nature (that is, In Control makes new versions of its tools and models available to all members to implement as they are developed, constantly seeking feedback and developing new, improved versions – much the same as IT companies issue new versions of their software). In one sense, therefore, In

Control might best be described as a 'social innovation network', seeking to connect key people together, develop new ideas, test them in practice and refine them over time. It also saw itself very much as 'a think tank that does' (personal communication), generating bottom–up solutions that build on the realities of the lives of service users, their families and front-line staff.

Box 5.2: The origins of In Control

In 2003 discussions [about how to transform the social care system] ... took place between Steve Jones, then Chief Executive of Wigan Metropolitan Borough Council, Martin Routledge of the Valuing People Support Team (VPST) and Julie Stansfield of the North West Training and Development Team. The emerging project gained strong support from Rob Greig, then leader of the VPST, and Jo Williams, Chief Executive of Mencap.

The group also included Helen Sanderson, one of the leading thinkers and practitioners of person-centred planning, and Simon Duffy of Paradigm (a leading consultancy agency). Simon Duffy had been working on practical systems for individualising funding so that individuals had more control of money for their support since the early 1990s. During this time he worked with service providers like Southwark Consortium and Inclusion Glasgow, and latterly with North Lanarkshire Council.

Carl Poll also joined the team. He was the founder of KeyRing, an innovative community support organisation ...

By late 2003, under the joint leadership of Mencap and VPST, the In Control Partnership was born ...

Aided by the sponsorship of the VPST and Mencap (each contributed £60,000), In Control was able to invite local authorities to participate in testing and further developing the model. Essex, Gateshead, Redcar and Cleveland, South Gloucestershire, West Sussex and Wigan came forward as the pilot authorities. Each authority contributed both funding (£20,000 each) and a commitment to building a new system of social care in their areas.

(Poll et al, 2006, p 8)

From here, it is harder to explain how the initial concept of personal budgets came to be taken up by government and promoted with such enthusiasm. Although it is beyond the scope of this book, the broader literature on policy making suggests that the way in which ideas are developed, announced and implemented can often be a form of 'muddling through' (Lindblom, 1959), based on an interaction between multiple and often competing interests. Certainly this seems to have been the case with the increasing policy interest in personal budgets. At this time, adult social care services were facing increasing pressure as a result of demographic and social changes, medical and technological advances and rising public expectations. Moreover, different interest groups appeared to have different motivations, with some interested in the potential of personal budgets to improve choice and control, and others seemingly interested more in whether this way of working could lead to cost savings (or at the very least make existing scarce resources go farther). In many ways, this seems similar to the history of direct payments, with different supporters potentially motivated by a desire to promote citizenship and independence, on the one hand, or by a desire to roll back the boundaries of the welfare state, on the other. While these two groups might be uneasy bedfellows in the long-term, they tended to create a momentum for change in the short-term when their interests and ideas began to coalesce.

Box 5.3: Seven steps to self-directed support

Step 1 – set a personal budget: using In Control's resource allocation system (RAS), everyone is told their financial allocation – their personal budget – and they decide what level of control they wish to take over their budget.

Step 2 – plan support: people plan how they will use their personal budget to get the help that is best for them; if they need help to plan, then advocates, brokers or others can support them.

Step 3 – agree plan: the local authority helps people to create good support plans, checks they are safe and makes sure that people have any necessary representation.

Step 4 – manage personal budget: people control their personal budget to the extent they want (there are currently six distinct degrees of control: ranging from direct payments at one extreme to local authority control at the other).

Step 5 – organise support: people can use their personal budget flexibly (including for statutory services). Indeed, the only real restriction is that the budget must be used for needs the state recognises as legitimate and must be spent on something legal.

Step 6 – live life: people use their personal budget to achieve the outcomes that are important to them in the context of their whole life and their role and contribution within the wider community.

Step 7 – review and learn: the authority continues to check that people are okay, shares what is being learned and can change things if people are not achieving the outcomes they need to achieve.

(Adapted from www.in-control.org.uk; see also Poll et al, 2006, pp 26–37)

While the exact factors that contributed to an expansion of personal budgets are likely to be unclear for some time, the fact remains that this was a new idea that looked good, that fitted with current policy aspirations and that seemed to work (see Chapter Six for further discussion of the development of policy from pilot projects). As Chris Hatton (2015) suggests in a fascinating review of work by Katherine Smith (2013), ideas that translate into policy often have to be consistent with (or capable of appearing consistent with) broader ideas held by government, have broad coalitions, be able to articulate a positive alternative (rather than just criticising existing arrangements) and have an already established institutional structure within government within which the idea can be readily embedded. While ideas that challenge the status quo without presenting a positive alternative are unlikely to be adopted, there are 'some ideas that are so flexible that they can be made to fit almost any set of government priorities'. Although charismatic ideas that fundamentally change current approaches can sometimes come along, they are rare. Perhaps in personal budgets we have a mix of charismatic ideas, flexibility and most of the policy prerequisites needed for an idea to be taken up. As Andrew Rowe suggested about direct payments in Chapter Three, perhaps this was simply 'an idea whose time had long since come'.

In 2005, official support for personal budgets came in three separate (albeit partially linked) government reports: the adult social care Green Paper, *Independence, Well-being and Choice*; a report from the Prime Minister's Strategy Unit on *Improving the Life Chances of Disabled People*; and a report from the Department for Work and Pensions, *Opportunity Age*, on the government's strategy for older people (see Box 5.4). Following this, a commitment to piloting personal budgets also appeared in the 2005 Labour Party manifesto. As explained below, however, the government often adopted the term 'individual budget' to refer to a broader, but less well-defined, notion of a personal budget made up with money from diverse funding sources.

Arising out of this, the government began a two-year pilot in 13 sites (see Table 5.1). Despite good intentions, this process seems to have struggled from something of an initial lack of clarity and from confusion over the key differences between the approaches being tested by In Control and DH. That this was the case seems to be demonstrated in a number of key early developments.

- The terminology used was confusing, with In Control and DH using the same term (which the former had invented) to refer to different concepts (see Box 5.5 for further discussion). While In Control initially used the term 'individual budget' to refer to its work in adult social care, DH used the same language to refer to a more integrated approach in which local pilots experimented with bringing together a series of different funding streams. In a later attempt to resolve this issue, DH began to refer to 'personal budgets' for approaches that involve adult social care only, and 'individual budgets' for approaches that seek to integrate multiple funding sources. Given the confusion that occurred when the Department for Work and Pensions

Box 5.4: Official interest in personal budgets

In 2005, the Department of Health's adult social care Green Paper, *Independence, Well-being and Choice*, proposed a series of pilots to develop the evidence base. Working with a number of different adult user groups and including a series of different budgets (including adult social care, equipment and adaptations, Independent Living Funds, Access to Work and Family Funds), the pilots (if successful) were expected to lead to the more widespread roll-out of personal budgets by 2012.

Also in 2005, the Prime Minister's Strategy Unit report on *Improving the Life Chances of Disabled People* argued that 'different sources of funding should be brought together in the form of individual budgets – while giving individuals the choice whether to take these budgets as cash or as services' (p 93). With national roll-out by 2012, this was to be based on a simplified resource allocation system, 'one-stop' assessment, greater self-assessment and access to advocacy.

This was supplemented by the Department for Work and Pensions report, *Opportunity Age*, which stated that 'we want to achieve a society where increasingly diverse older people are active consumers of public services, exercising choice and control, not passive recipients of them ... Over the next years, we will test out services which implement this model ..., including giving those who want them individual budgets which they can use to select their own care packages' (DWP, 2005, p xviii).

Finally, in 2005, the Labour Party manifesto pledged to 'give older people greater choice over their care. For every older person receiving care or other support, we want to offer transparent, individual budgets which bring funding for a range of services ... together in one place. We will pilot individual budgets for older people by the end of this year' (p 72).

developed a new policy for the 'direct payment' of social security benefits (see Chapter Three), this seemed an unfortunate case of history repeating itself. Perhaps more importantly, it also meant that the national IBSEN evaluation of individual budgets, described in more detail below, was actually exploring something different to the model of self-directed support developed by In Control, and results therefore need to be interpreted with caution (see Chapter Six for further discussion).

- After its initial pilot work in six local authorities, In Control began a second phase of work in late 2005 – within three months it had some 60 local authorities sign up as members. However, several of DH's 13 pilot sites were also In Control members (and indeed a small number of authorities were members of the original In Control six, the 60 Phase 2 projects and DH pilots).

- The focus of the initial DH approach was on integrating locally a series of relatively small-scale but very bureaucratic funding sources. While some progress was made, this seemed to set local pilots up to fail by asking them to tackle systemic issues that needed national attention (and perhaps even new legislation). Arguably, this was the wrong tactic to be adopting; perhaps greater progress could have been made by focusing on the much larger adult social care budget, rather than diluting the In Control model by taking on too many different funding sources at once.

- With the benefit of hindsight, DH pilots seemed to suffer early on from a lack of clarity about the nature of the intervention that was being tested, tight timescales, strong political interest and the difficulty of establishing cross–government pilots.

Table 5.1: DH individual budget pilot sites

Site	Main focus
Gateshead	People with learning difficulties, people with physical/sensory impairments and people with mental health problems at times of transition from children's services to adult services, and from adult services to older people's services
Coventry	People with learning difficulties, people with physical/sensory impairments and people who use mental health services. They will all be people who are going through changes in their lives – e.g. growing up, moving from education to employment, leaving a family or other 'supervised' home to live more independently, moving from hospital or rehab to living in the community or at home, and people who are coming home from living in an 'out of city' placement.
West Sussex	Older people
Manchester	Older people, people with neurological illness, renal patients
Oldham	All adults
Barnsley	All adults, including young people in transition
Lincolnshire	Starting with older people, but later to include all adults
Barking and Dagenham	Older people, people with learning difficulties, people with physical impairments and people who use mental health services
Kensington and Chelsea	Older people and people with physical impairments
Leicester	People with learning difficulties, people with physical/sensory impairments. May include other people later in the pilot
Bath and North East Somerset	People with learning difficulties, older people and younger people with a physical/sensory impairment
Essex	People with learning difficulties, people with physical impairments, family carers
Norfolk	People with mental health problems

Source: Care Services Improvement Partnership individual budget website (http://individualbudgets.csip.org.uk/dynamic/dohpage2.jsp, accessed 20 June 2008).

> **Box 5.5: Changing language**
>
> Over time, the language used to describe this area of policy and practice has changed – and not always helpfully. Risking complicating matters yet further, a brief history is set out below. When the initial group of people met in 2003 to share ideas, the term initially used was 'self-directed services'. However, it very quickly became apparent that this was not quite right (because it focused too much on formal services), and so the shorthand term was changed to 'self-directed support'. Also at this time, the individuals involved decided that they needed a name and a brand for what they were starting to try to create, and chose 'In Control'.
>
> By 2004, members of In Control were talking about the importance of an 'indicative resource allocation' (which, for some reason, never caught on!). Initially it is believed to have been a government minister who started using the term 'individual budget' to provide a more helpful summary of the concept (and certainly one that flows off the tongue better).
>
> Following government interest in using this model to integrate different funding streams, the Department of Health and others began to reserve the term 'individual budget' to refer to the range of different models that they were piloting (see Table 5.1). In Control was therefore asked to find another term for its work in adult social care, deciding upon 'personal budgets' as an appropriate compromise. It therefore had to rewrite all its material, replacing 'individual budgets' with 'personal budgets'.
>
> In response to these complexities, this book tries to use the term 'personal budget' to refer to the work of In Control and to changes in adult social care, reserving the term 'individual budget' for initial Department of Health pilots involving the integration of multiple funding sources.

In spite of their very promising start and fairly unpromising national adoption, policy remained committed to the potential of personal budgets. That this was the case seems, at least in part, to owe something to the personal contribution of Ivan Lewis, then the care services minister, who became very much a champion of In Control and personal budgets. Thus, in late 2007, the government's *Putting People First* manifesto (HM Government, 2007) was signed by six government departments and a series of national health, social care and local government organisations (see Box 5.6). Although the self-proclaimed 'shared vision and commitment to the transformation of adult social care' set out a number of different approaches, the document pledged a further increase in the number of direct payment recipients as well as 'personal budgets for everyone eligible for publicly funded adult social care support other than in circumstances where people require emergency access to provision' (HM Government, 2007, p 3). At the same time, there was also a suggestion that 'in the future personal budgets for people with long-term conditions could include NHS resources' (HM Government, 2007, p 3). In early 2008, this was followed by a more detailed circular that focused more on implementation and support, including a new three-year £520 million grant to help councils make the necessary changes (DH,

2008a). Increasingly, these reforms were described in terms of a 'personalisation agenda', in which 'every person across the spectrum of need [has] choice and control over the shape of his or her support, in the most appropriate setting' (DH, 2008a, p 2). While on one hand this seemed like a reasonable shorthand for a more complex and important series of changes, it arguably lacked much of the clarity and practical focus of In Control's notion of 'self-directed support'.

As a result of these developments, personal budgets seemed set to transform the nature of adult social care, and the numbers of people involved increased rapidly. From six pilots and 60 people receiving personal budgets from late 2003, In Control had achieved a membership of 108 local authorities by late 2008, by which time an estimated 3,500 people across the UK were receiving personal budgets (Hatton et al, 2008, p 2). In addition, 19 sites had committed to a rapid and widespread implementation of personal budgets, known as 'total transformation' (committing to 50% of all service users receiving a personal budget within three years), while additional projects around 'Taking Control' (in children's services) and 'Staying in Control' (in health) had 27 children's departments and 37 NHS members respectively.

Box 5.6: *Putting People First*

Ensuring older people, people with chronic conditions, disabled people and people with mental health problems have the best possible quality of life and the equality of independent living is fundamental to a socially just society. For many, social care is the support which helps make this a reality ... The time has now come to build on best practice and replace paternalistic, reactive care of variable quality with a mainstream system focused on prevention, early intervention, enablement, and high quality personally tailored services. In the future, we want people to have the maximum choice, control and power over the support services they receive.

(HM Government, 2007, p 2)

Key features, concepts and values

Given criticisms about the poorly explained nature of personal budgets at national level, it is important to be clear about the key features of this way of working. As personal budgets became something of a hot topic, the biggest danger was that they would get hijacked by people who did not understand them or who had other motives, allowing the old system to pay lip-service to the concept while essentially recreating itself. To guard against this, In Control set out seven key principles (Hatton et al, 2008, pp 3–4).

- *The right to independent living*: if someone has an impairment that means they need help to fulfil their needs as a citizen, they should get the help they need.

- *Right to a personal budget*: if someone needs ongoing paid help as part of their life, they should be able to decide how the money that pays for that help is used.
- *Right to self-determination*: if someone needs help to make decisions, then decision making should be made as close to the person as possible, reflecting the person's own interests and preferences.
- *Right to accessibility*: the system of rules within which people have to work must be clear and open in order to maximise the ability of people to take control of their own support.
- *Right to flexible funding*: when someone is using their personal budget they should be free to spend their funds in the way that makes best sense to them, without unnecessary restrictions.
- *Accountability principle*: the person and the government both have a responsibility to each other to explain their decisions and to share what they have learnt.
- *Capacity principle*: people, their families and communities must not be assumed to be incapable of managing their own support, learning skills or making a contribution.

Building on this, In Control characterised its approach as shifting from a 'professional gift' model (in which the state uses the money it receives from taxes to slot people into pre-paid services through the work of professional assessors and gatekeepers) to a 'citizenship model' (in which the disabled person is at the centre of the process, is part of the community and organises the support they need and want; see Figures 5.1 and 5.2). While personal budgets are important, therefore, it is this shift in the relationship between the state and the individual that lies at the heart of self-directed support. This is also helpfully captured by Rummery (2006, pp 646–7), who argues that:

> The problem is that community care policy has never been framed within a discourse of citizenship ... New Labour has left largely unchallenged a system of providing care and support for disabled people that was designed by the Conservative government to curb the spiralling cost of residential care provision and marketise the delivery of welfare. The fundamental aims and discourse of community care policy need to be challenged. We need to stop talking about 'the cost of care' and start talking about supporting citizenship and challenging social exclusion.

In developing this further, In Control summarised some of the key differences between traditional approaches to social care and the new system of self-directed support (see Table 5.2).

Table 5.2: Social care versus self-directed support

Beliefs for social care	Beliefs for self-directed support
Disabled people are vulnerable and should be taken care of by trained professionals	Every adult should be in control of their life, even if they need help with decisions
Existing services suit people well – the challenge is to assess people and decide which service suits them	Everybody needs support that is tailored to their situation to help them sustain and build their place in the community
Money is not abused if it is controlled by large organisations or statutory authorities	Money is most likely to be used well when it is controlled by the person or by people who really care about the person
Family and friends are unreliable allies for disabled people and where possible should be replaced by independent professionals	Family and friends can be the most important allies for disabled people and make a positive contribution to their lives

Source: Duffy, 2005b, p 10.

Figure 5.1: Professional gift model of social care

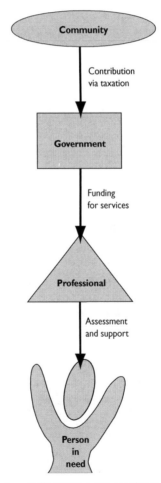

Reproduced with permission from Duffy, 2005c, p 153; see also Duffy, 1996.

Figure 5.2: Citizenship model

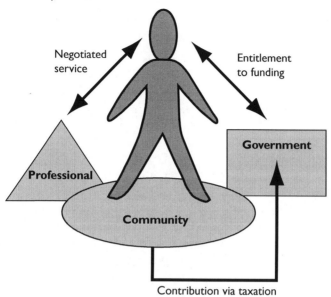

Once a system of self-directed support is in place, it should include the seven steps set out previously in Box 5.3 (p 73). While these are relatively self-explanatory, five particular issues are worthy of further exploration:

- Philosophically, personal budgets and self-directed support link naturally to notions of self-assessment and person-centred planning. These are complex and important issues, and further details and resources are available via www. in-control.org.uk.
- Following an assessment, the person is effectively placed in a funding bracket according to the level of their needs using a Resource Allocation System (RAS). While this is an issue that often concerns local authorities, In Control undertook significant work developing and improving the RAS process (see Box 5.7 for a brief summary). Crucially, the RAS was only ever intended to be indicative – giving people a quick and easy sense of the levels of funding likely to be available with which to plan, but not being set in stone. With hindsight, of course, it is perhaps unsurprising that many councils appear to have struggled to retain this degree of flexibility in practice (see Chapter Six for further discussion).
- Next is the centrality of the Support Plan, which should be done wherever possible by the person themselves and anyone else they wish to be involved (often friends and family). However, there are many other forms of support that should be available, including different forms of advice and brokerage (see Tables 5.3 and 5.4). A helpful overview is provided by Senker (2008), who summarises the tasks or functions that underpin the notion of 'support

brokerage' and sets out practical examples and ideas to help develop this. In some ways, this broader notion of brokerage may contrast with the strong emphasis on CILs in the development of direct payments. Although support for personal budgets may well come from a CIL, there is no assumption that this is necessarily the optimal solution. Indeed, in an era when we no longer block-purchase care on people's behalf, it seems ironic to be block-purchasing support for people (albeit that councils should, in our view, be supporting CILs on principle so that there are vibrant user-led organisations locally).

• After this, the management of a personal budget can be undertaken by a range of different people, depending on the needs and wishes of the person concerned (see Table 5.3). This again seems different from direct payments, where some local authorities seemed to adopt a 'take it or leave it' approach: if you were perceived as not liking what the local authority was offering, then you were on your own (see, for example, Sapey and Pearson, 2004). A particularly interesting option here is the 'individual service fund', with personal budget holders choosing to work together with a trusted service provider on how the money is spent over time (see Sanderson and Miller, 2014 for an introduction). Unfortunately, this option remains under-developed and this seems something of a missed opportunity (see Chapter Six).

• In contrast to traditional social care, the emphasis shifts from the initial assessment (which often dominates much of current practice) to support planning and review (which are often neglected when workloads are heavy). In many ways, this reverses current practice, and is arguably a better place to focus in order to ensure the best possible support arrangements and the maximum possible learning.

Emerging evidence about impact

From the relatively humble origins described above, In Control conducted a brief evaluation of the impact of self-directed support on the lives of a very small sample of people (31) in the first six pilot sites (see Poll et al, 2006 for all findings quoted in this and the next two paragraphs). Overseen by Professor Chris Hatton from the University of Lancaster, the evaluation involved before and after questionnaires completed by the individuals concerned (with an average of 46 weeks between the first and second questionnaires, range 18–61 weeks). Although only based on a very small group of people, the findings were so encouraging that they generated debate and enthusiasm above and beyond the numbers involved. At the same time, it should be remembered that this sample was not necessarily representative and that many people who volunteer for pilots can sometimes be those who are the most dissatisfied with current arrangements and/or with the most motivation to make new approaches work. In addition, we have no information on what would have happened to these individuals anyway without the pilot, and so the relationship between the outcomes below and the

Box 5.7: The history of the RAS

RAS Version 1 – The first version of the RAS was developed by Simon Duffy before the beginning of In Control and it involved setting the budget in the light of three criteria: need, complexity, and community support ...

RAS Version 2 – At the beginning of In Control's early work in Wigan in 2003, Simon worked with colleagues to develop a more sophisticated system. This system set personal budget levels by correlating them to the cost of typical existing service packages ...

RAS Version 3 – In 2005, John Walters joined In Control as its technical director and brought with him a more sophisticated model of needs analysis that allowed the model to put a numeric value on different domains of need ...

RAS Version 4 – In 2006, more authorities wanted a system that could cope with much higher numbers of people from different care groups. John developed a new approach that allowed authorities to apply a 'price point' that would be multiplied by the figure that represented the level of need ...

RAS Version 5 – In 2007, John began work with [In Control's] partner organisation, Symmetric SD, to develop a further version of the RAS that could be delivered through the internet. This is called e-RAS. The key innovation here has been that In Control is finally able to go beyond setting the personal budget level by reference to the cost profile of the past. Instead, it is possible to use the data that is coming from the field to set the budget level.

(Hatton et al, 2008, p 35)

Since then, a number of commentators feel that the RAS has become too complicated in many councils – a barrier to change rather than a simple tool to help people plan (see Chapter Six for further discussion).

concept of a personal budget is not necessarily causal. That said, the results are so promising that they remain worthy of further study.

As Table 5.5 suggests, at the second questionnaire more people felt that they were making the important decisions over their own lives and were in control of their money. Satisfaction with support also increased (from 48% to 100%). Perhaps most important of all, many of the people involved were able to make significant changes in their lives (see Tables 5.6–5.7), shifting away from more institutional forms of support to more community-based, personalised ways of meeting need. In particular, the ten people living in residential care at the start of the process were all able to move into alternative accommodation in under a year. More generally, people made greater use of PAs and community support, with less use of services such as day care.

Table 5.3: Different types of support

Source of support	
The person themselves, their friends and family	Wherever possible, this should be the main source of support
Support brokers	Help from an independent source – someone who is not involved in either arranging or providing support
Service providers	Help from a service provider the person trusts
Care managers	Some people may still need help from care managers – but a system of self-directed support should free them up from doing this for everyone in order to concentrate on those with the most complex needs and without access to other support
People in the community	Brokerage consists of a set of functions that could be carried out by many other people – including individuals, family members and community organisations

Source: Poll et al, 2006, p 31.

Table 5.4: Managing a personal budget

Disabled person	The person manages their own money and support
Representative	A representative manages on the person's behalf
Trust	A trust is established to receive and control the money on the person's behalf (similar to a trust that might be set up for a child who inherits money)
Broker	Some people choose to pay an individual or organisation to act as their broker
Service provider	The service provider manages the person's money, but keeps it separate in an Individual Service Fund and spends it on behalf of/with the individual
Care manager	Some people may still want or need their care manager to manage their personal budget on their behalf

Source: Poll et al, 2006, p 33.

Table 5.5: The impact of personal budgets (2006)

Impact of personal budgets	Number of people (at Time 1 and Time 2) (total n = 31)
Making important decisions about your life	Doubled (from 6 to 12)
Control over your life	Increased from no one really happy to 17 really happy
Person-centred plan	Numbers with a plan increased from 12 to 27
Satisfaction with support	Went from 6 really unhappy and 9 unhappy to no one really unhappy or unhappy
Satisfaction with the money you have	From 9 really unhappy/7 unhappy/12 quite happy/2 really happy to 1/1/15/13 respectively
Happy with your home	From 10 really happy to 23 really happy
Happy with relationships	Most were at least fairly happy before, but there was still an improvement

Adapted from Poll et al, 2006.

Table 5.6 Changes in people's lives

Desired change	% achieved
Where I live	76%
Who I live with	81%
What I do with my time	69%
Who supports me	89%

Source: Poll et al, 2006, p 52.

Table 5.7: Type of support

Type of support	Before	After
Support at home	20	22
Employing PAs	8	22
Using day centre	12	11
Hours in day centre	4.5 days	3.5 days
Using family support	21	21
Using community support	8	15

Source: Poll et al, 2006, p 81.

Also significant was the impact on the cost of current support packages. While all the above caveats about the size and limitations of the sample still apply, work in five other local authorities resulted in significant savings (the smallest amount saved was 12%; see Table 5.8). In the view of In Control, this was largely due to a more transparent allocation system that cut out expensive outlying cases and to a natural tendency for block-purchased services to over-provide even for people with lower levels of need (that is, once a service is block-purchased, it tends to get used, irrespective of whether the individual really needs it or not). Although this issue is explored in more detail in Chapter Seven, these early findings clearly made an important impact on some policy makers and local authority leaders: based on the initial evaluation (albeit very small and limited), personal budgets seemed to hold out the possibility of achieving much better outcomes for less money, and few could ignore such a potential holy grail.

Table 5.8: The impact of personal budgets on costs

Authority	Sum of support pre-In Control (£)	Sum of personal budgets (£)	Difference (%)
1	600,000	525,000	12
2 (desk exercise)	5,625,000	4,500,000	20
3 (in cases where there was a difference)	194,000	107,000	45
4	187,305	152,300	19
5	594,000	397,000	33

Source: Poll et al, 2006, p 67.

In 2007, Henwood and Hudson (2007b) published findings from a Department of Health-funded review of early progress with self-directed support in three case study localities. These were deliberately chosen to include a spectrum of experiences, with one site an In Control pilot, one aiming to move towards large-scale transformation and one having had little engagement with self-directed support. Although at this stage there was little evidence about the impact of self-directed support on people's lives, the review provided a helpful snapshot of the implementation of this new way of working and identified a series of practical and cultural issues that would need to be overcome (see Chapters Seven and Eight).

By 2008, Poll et al's (2006) evaluation was supplemented by more detailed research based on interviews with 196 people using self-directed support in 17 local authorities across England (Hatton et al, 2008). Again overseen by Professor Chris Hatton, the evaluation was at pains to stress the potential limitations of the study (for example, it was an incomplete and not necessarily representative sample, and people with learning difficulties and with physical impairments were more likely to report improvements than the small number of older people who took part). However, the fact remains that self-directed support again seemed to lead to positive outcomes (see Box 5.8), including significant improvements in some people's health and well-being, time spent with people they liked, quality of life, choice and control, contributions to community life and personal dignity.

Box 5.8: Outcomes of self-directed support (2008)

Participants reported improvement in:

Quality of life (76%)
Choice and control (72%)
Taking part in and contributing to the community (64%)
Personal dignity (59%)
Spending time with people you like (55%)
Health and well-being (47%)
Economic well-being (36%)
Feeling safe and secure at home (29%)

Of the 196 participants, 58% were people with learning difficulties, 20% were people with physical impairments and 13% were older people. 89% were White, 8% Asian and 4% Black. For some outcomes, people with learning difficulties and people with physical impairments were more likely to report improvement than older people (although this may be because the small numbers of older people involved were less likely to have been using services before the introduction of self-directed support and had, on average, used self-directed support for a shorter period of time).

(Hatton et al, 2008)

Although this book has so far tended to focus on the needs of adults, personal budgets have significant implications for disabled children, for young people with support needs and for children's services more generally. This is a complex area, but a chapter by Nic Crosby in the 2008 summary of In Control's second phase provides a helpful overview (see Box 5.9). Essentially, Crosby's chapter argues that self-directed support should start as soon as people need additional support, whether this is at birth, on going to school, on moving into secondary education or on entering adulthood. From early initiatives in this field, it appears as though there are significant potential benefits to families taking greater control over the support that is provided to young children with support needs and that such ways of working could also help to ease transition into adult life.

Box 5.9: Children and families in control

As summarised by Crosby (2008, p 79), key early initiatives included:

- *Dynamite*: a two-year programme led by Paradigm to develop a model of self-directed support for young people.
- *Person-centred transition review*: a series of Valuing People Support Team pilots.
- *Improving Choice*: a programme by the Eastern Region Learning and Skills Council to use 'transition brokers' to develop post-16 provision for young people with learning difficulties who would otherwise have to attend specialist residential colleges.
- *Budget-holding lead professionals*: government pilot to explore how lead professionals can hold a small budget on behalf of individual children and families (see also Office for Public Management, 2006).
- *Learning and Living Now*: Mencap project to support young people with learning difficulties. This includes a resource-allocation system, learning and living support plans and personalised support.
- *Building Blocks*: a project in Devon and Cornwall to explain concepts of choice, decision making and taking control.
- *Person-centred Curriculum*: to support children and young people to develop the skills and approaches for self-directed futures.
- *Taking Control*: In Control's programme for children and young people, beginning with eight children's services in Autumn 2007.

As part of a separate process, DH commissioned researchers from the universities of York, Manchester, Kent, King's College London and the London School of Economics to carry out an independent evaluation of the 13 Department of Health pilot sites (that is, sites integrating other funding streams above and beyond adult social care). Published in the autumn of 2008, the final report (Glendinning et al, 2008, known as the IBSEN study) was 305 pages in length and provided an important insight into the early impact of individual budgets. To reiterate a point made earlier in this chapter, the DH pilots were very different in origin and focus from the concept of self-directed support developed and evaluated by In Control – although many of the findings from IBSEN are relevant to both DH pilots and In Control. Given the scale and breadth of IBSEN, moreover, a more complex and nuanced picture was always likely to emerge than was the case in earlier and more pragmatic evaluations. As suggested above, the advent of self-directed support has the potential to change the whole of the adult social care system, and any national evaluation was always likely to find a mix of positives, negatives, enablers and barriers. Indeed, if we carried out a national evaluation of the current system, the result would probably be equally complex, mixed and difficult to interpret. Finally, any national evaluation was always bound to struggle with trying to unpick which barriers and challenges are inherent to the concept of individual budgets, and which are more to do with the nature of pilot projects more generally. As a result, there was always likely to be a risk of mixed messages when the final IBSEN evaluation was published, and supporters and critics alike are likely to find much in the final report to debate and to reflect on in more detail.

With these caveats in mind, IBSEN remains crucial. Conducted by a series of leading social policy and social work researchers, the final study is detailed, rigorous and extremely rich in terms of the data it provides. Although key messages are summarised in Box 5.10, the research is so in-depth that it deserves careful study in its own right (and the very brief overview provided here cannot do justice to such a complex evaluation). The study was also conducted in tight timescales, with significant political interest and a number of policy changes and delays – so much so that the researchers are to be congratulated for having been able to produce such a detailed insight in such difficult circumstances. Running from April 2006 to March 2008, the research focused on the outcomes of individual budgets, the experience of different user groups, factors aiding/hindering implementation and issues of effectiveness and cost-effectiveness. While the exact approach adopted is summarised in detail in the report itself, the research was based on a range of methods, including interviews with service users, front-line staff, local managers and individual budget leads, as well as a randomised controlled trial (an approach that allowed the researchers to compare costs and outcomes for people receiving an individual budget with those of a comparison group).

Given its complexity, IBSEN was accompanied by a DH summary (2008b), setting out key findings and providing an overview of the DH's response. Essentially, the DH interpreted IBSEN as demonstrating that individual budgets can lead to better outcomes and higher perceived levels of control, with particular benefits for people with mental health problems. Perhaps unsurprisingly, the DH's response spends significant time on the barriers that seem to exist within older people's services, and a linked report (DH, 2008c) summarises emerging lessons about good practice in this crucial area. Although some would see this as an attempt to put a positive gloss on a more nuanced set of findings, the DH's analysis of the current challenges in older people's services seems to us to be a helpful summary (DH, 2008c, p 1):

Previous experience with direct payments suggested that there would be significant challenges in making individual budgets work well for older people, particularly given the timescales of the [DH pilots]. The personalised approach of self-directed support represents a profound shift in focus; instead of being passive recipients of services, older people become active participants in their care and support. The experience of implementing individualised funding is less developed for older people than for younger disabled adults. This meant there was less experience to build on for older people and professionals working with them.

Box 5.10: The national IBSEN evaluation

- Overall, the study found 'encouraging indications of the impact of IBs [individual budgets] on individuals' lives, particularly the fact that those receiving IBs felt more in control of their lives than the comparison group' (p 236).
- Individual budgets are at least cost neutral – indeed they seem to cost on average £279 per week, as compared to £296 for standard services (although this difference was not statistically significant).
- In the short term at least, there was evidence to suggest that supporting people to access individual budgets may take additional staff time – and it remains to be seen whether this will reduce in future as the pilots are mainstreamed.
- Individual budgets had particular benefits for people with mental health problems and younger disabled people, with mixed results for people with learning difficulties.
- However, results were much less positive for older people, with the researchers pointing to a number of potential contributing factors (such as anxiety about potential changes to established support, fears about the burden of greater control, a tendency to approach services only in a crisis, the focus of older people's services on meeting personal care needs rather than broader elements of well-being, and the tendency for older people to receive smaller care packages, as compared to younger disabled people).
- Despite support for the potential to integrate different funding sources, this was a major source of frustration at a local level with only limited progress (as many of the funding streams arguably require national action if they are to be successfully integrated).

For further discussion of key enablers and barriers (including the impact on front-line staff; issues of eligibility, assessment and resource allocation; support planning and brokerage; risk; the experience of providers and commissioners; and the relationship with the NHS), see the full report (Glendinning et al, 2008). The final study also contains a wealth of information on people's hopes and aspirations, how they spent their budgets and the views of front-line staff.

SUMMARY

Having summarised the history, spread and key features of personal budgets, this chapter has set out the (impressive) results of early research and evaluation of these small-scale pilot projects. While the very real limitations of these emerging findings were recognised, the positives that were achieved were so significant that the concept of personal budgets was taken up by policy makers and quickly became a cornerstone of adult social care reform. Building on the contribution of direct payments, personal budgets and self-directed support offer an even broader approach that seeks to transform the adult social care system as a whole. As these ideas were picked up by government, the subsequent national pilots ran the risk of blurring the initial clarity of the In Control model, perhaps signalling the risks that can occur when new ideas are rolled out nationally at pace and scale (see Chapter Six). This was a clear finding of the IBSEN study, which revealed significant positives, but also numerous challenges in terms of implementation, a potential lack of clarity around key concepts in some quarters and a mixed experience for some user groups. Nonetheless, personal budgets had already been picked up by national policy makers with enthusiasm, and the publication of IBSEN marked their arrival in mainstream policy and practice.

IMPLICATIONS FOR POLICY AND PRACTICE

- By being clear with people from the outset how much money is available to plan their support there is scope for people to be much more innovative. They can also go about meeting needs in a way that makes sense to them, given their individual circumstances and aspirations.
- Viewed from this angle, personal budgets are nothing more than 'sensible delegation', and the assumption is that the best person to make decisions about support is often the person with support needs themselves or someone as close to them as possible.
- Although there are practical and cultural issues to overcome, personal budgets seem to have had extremely positive results in terms of outcomes for people needing support and effective use of scarce public resources.
- Personal budgets give a greater sense of transparency and citizen entitlement. In this sense, they represent a shift in the relationship between the individual and the state that could have implications for a number of other public services.
- While the government is to be commended for recognising the benefits of personal budgets and committing to rolling them out, there is a very real risk that a lack of understanding of the underlying principles of self-directed support could significantly limit the impact of personal budgets.

RECOMMENDED READING AND USEFUL WEBSITES

For further details on the nature and impact of personal/individual budgets, see:

- early In Control evaluations (Poll et al, 2006; Hatton et al, 2008);
- Henwood and Hudson's (2007b) report on the implementation of self-directed support;
- the final report of IBSEN (Glendinning et al, 2008) – in addition to the full study, a series of early articles shed light on some of the emerging challenges (Manthorpe et al, 2009a–b; Rabiee et al, 2009), while two DH reports (2008b–c) explore next steps and emerging good practice in older people's services.

Useful introductions are also available in Simon Duffy's articles in *Journal of Integrated Care* (e.g. Duffy, 2004, 2005a, 2006, 2007), while Demos provides an overview that is free to download (Leadbeater et al, 2008 – see www.demos.co.uk).

Official policy aspirations are set out in *Putting People First* (HM Government, 2007) and the more detailed local authority circular on *Transforming Social Care* (DH, 2008a). Earlier documents such as the social care Green Paper (DH, 2005) and *Improving the Life Chances of Disabled People* (Prime Minister's Strategy Unit, 2005) are also useful. For an overview, SCIE (2008) publishes a 'rough guide' to personalisation.

For personal accounts, good practice examples and access to relevant documents, processes and templates, see the In Control website (www.in-control.org.uk) or that of the Centre for Welfare Reform (www.centreforwelfrereform.org). The *Living Your Life, Your Way* DVD (Department of Health/Care Services Improvement Partnership/In Control, 2008) also provides a series of personal accounts of the practicalities, the power and the potential impact of personal budgets.

While much of this book tends to focus on the implications for disabled people and for front-line staff, there are clearly significant implications for current commissioners and service providers (see, for example, Tyson, nd; OPM, 2007; Baxter et al, 2008; Bennett, 2008; CSIP, 2008; Glendinning et al, 2008 for early discussion).

REFLECTIVE EXERCISES

1. This is an area of policy and practice that is rarely explained well. Having read this chapter, make sure that you are confident about how you would define a personal budget and its potential benefits. Practise explaining this to others and see how easy or otherwise it is to answer their questions.

2. We often demand higher standards of proof for new ways of working than we do for previous approaches, and place new ideas under greater scrutiny than the status quo. Write a list of the pros and cons of direct services, of direct payments and of personal budgets.

3. Think of someone you know with social care needs. What impact might personal budgets have for them?

4. Look at the website of your local council. How does this explain personal budgets, and to what extent is this consistent with some of the history and principles set out in this chapter?

5. Think about what is important to you in your everyday life. If you had social care needs would you want a personal budget, and how might it compare to direct services?

SIX

The lessons of personal budgets – how they spread and what they achieved

This chapter explores:
- the mainstreaming of personal budgets from 2008 onwards;
- emerging evidence about impact now that we have greater experience of implementation;
- the experience of different user groups and different areas of the country;
- the potential implications for wider public services.

With hindsight, the speed with which the concept of personal budgets – initially developed and tested bottom-up through a series of small-scale local pilots – was taken up by policy makers is astounding. In a remarkably short period of time, personal budgets had been identified by the New Labour government as a key element of adult social care reform, and were increasingly seen as having potential for the reform of other public services as well. Moreover, there was significant cross-party consensus around the importance of personal budgets and the broader personalisation agenda, with the Conservative/Liberal Democrat Coalition government of 2010–15 effectively continuing where New Labour had left off. In particular, the Coalition continued to stress that all adult social care would be delivered via a personal budget and that this way of working had real potential for other areas of state welfare (particularly in health care). However, it also went a step further in setting out an expectation that all personal budgets would take the form of a direct payment:

> Where personalisation has taken root, it works and is popular with users and carers ... The time is now right to make personal budgets the norm for everyone who receives ongoing care and support – ideally as a direct cash payment, to give maximum flexibility and choice. (DH, 2010b, p 16)

While some people were nervous that this would mean people who might not want a direct payment being forced to have one, it is more likely that this was an attempt to shift the emphasis of recent debates. Whereas in some areas of the country it seemed as if many people would be given a local authority-managed budget (unless there was a good reason why not), this statement by the Coalition was arguably an attempt to ensure that most people would receive a direct payment (seen as a particularly strong form of choice and control) unless there was a good reason why not. In one sense, this continues previous policies where many adult social care service users initially received a direct service unless there was a good reason why not, until a potential tipping point was reached and personal budgets/direct payments became the norm. In time it is possible that the Coalition's intervention will achieve another such tipping point, with direct payments becoming the default option.

Mainstreaming personal budgets

In 2008, the publication of the national IBSEN study represented a key transition in the history of personal budgets (Glendinning et al, 2008). After emerging as a series of small-scale, bottom-up innovations in local authorities keen to test new approaches, this way of working had become national policy – and now had the research evidence to prove its potential impact. While all national evaluations involve positives, negatives, nuance and caveats, IBSEN was nevertheless seen by many as proof that personal budgets were here to stay. Rather than being a recent innovation or an 'add on' to the current system, personal budgets were now going to be 'the system'. Of course, moving from initial innovation with sites, staff and service users keen to experiment to an approach where the innovation becomes the new orthodoxy, implemented everywhere at pace and scale, is an incredibly risky transition. In particular, there is a danger that something important is lost in the process, that lip-service is paid to key underlying principles and/or that implementation happens piecemeal and with conflicting values and motives. For many people, personalisation was not at its most vulnerable when it was just developing and testing new approaches – but when it became national policy. An excellent blog by Gerald Wistow (2015), scientific advisor to the individual budgets team at the DH, provides a succinct summary of these developments, while also reflecting on the tensions that can arise between the policy process and academics involved in policy evaluations.

Since 2008, there have been additional studies confirming that personal budgets can be a positive experience for people previously using direct services and can improve outcomes. This includes data from ongoing monitoring by In Control and partners (see Box 6.1) as well as a second study by the IBSEN team, which found that personal budgets can also achieve positive outcomes for carers at no higher cost than conventional services (Glendinning et al, 2009). To help build on these early insights, a series of national social care bodies formed the Think Local Act Personal (TLAP, 2011a–b) partnership, seeking to support the implementation of personalisation and to transform the adult social care system (see www.thinklocalactpersonal.org.uk). TLAP has since become an important player in the spread of personal budgets, helping to make available a series of accessible publications around good practice, local experience, toolkits and other resources for areas keen to implement national policy as effectively as possible – but to do so in a way which really makes a positive difference for people using services (see further resources at the end of this chapter for more details). There has also been growing attention to the experience of other countries, seeking to learn potential lessons for the UK (see, for example, Carr and Robbins, 2009 for an early summary; see also Alakeson, 2010a; Gadsby et al, 2013; Grasser et al, 2013; Health Foundation, 2010, 2011 for international reviews around personal health budgets).

Box 6.1: Personal Budgets Outcomes and Evaluation Toolkit (POET)

In 2014, the third national personal budget survey (completed by 2,679 personal budget holders) found that:

- At least two-thirds of people said personal budgets had made things better or a lot better in 11 of 15 areas asked about – including dignity in support (82%), independence (78.9%), arranging support (79.9%), relationships with people paid to support them (75.9%) and quality of life (81.4%).
- More than two-thirds of carers said that things had got better or a lot better in terms of their ability to continue caring (78.6%), quality of life for the person being cared for (79.6%) and quality of life for the carer (71.3%).
- Fewer than 5% of people reported personal budgets having a negative impact on any of the 15 areas asked about.
- However, a number of people experienced difficulties with official systems and processes – summarised by the authors in terms of 'the challenges of uneven delivery and the continued experience of frustrating and unhelpful process' (p 74).

Summarised from Waters and Hatton (2014)

Implementing personal budgets in practice – growing unease and emerging tensions?

Alongside the primarily positive findings above, a number of studies and broader commentaries have also continued to emerge around potential limitations (see, for example, Slasberg et al, 2012a–b; Beresford, 2014a; see also Ridley et al, 2011 for evidence around the complexities of trying to implement self-directed support in Scotland). At times, these debates have become more than a little heated, to such an extent that we would argue that the vehemence of different stances might be to do with more than just the underlying data. As Needham and Glasby (2014, pp 16–17) have argued:

> Another contested element of personalisation is the extent to which it has been based on formal evidence, or rather has proceeded on the basis of anecdotal claims about its effectiveness. Certainly, there is no shortage of formal evaluation data about personalisation. The Department of Health (DH) funded a major evaluation of individual budgets (Glendinning et al, 2008) and has subsequently funded a

large-scale evaluation of personal health budgets (Forder et al, 2012). In Control run a national evaluation each year, using the Personal Budgets Outcome and Evaluation Tool (POET). ADASS undertake an annual survey on levels of take up of personal budgets. Community Care and Unison together have surveyed social work staff annually on their views of personalisation. Many other organisations have formally evaluated aspects of personalisation or undertaken evidence reviews to share best practice (e.g. the Social Care Institute for Excellence, the Audit Commission, the Cabinet Office, and the New Local Government Network).

However, concerns have been expressed about the extent to which personalisation has been promoted on the basis of a shallow evidence base. As Beresford (2011/12, p 37) puts it, 'The narrative of individual/personal budgets was then sold powerfully through stories from some service users of new flexibility and opportunities in their lives, far better than reliance on traditional services.' Individual testimonies have played a key role in establishing policy support for personalisation (Needham, 2011). As a member of In Control put it, '"One of the things that we did very early on was start to tell positive stories about self directed support and how it was working, and that's what's captured the imagination"' (cited in Needham, 2011).

It is possible to characterise diverse responses to the evidence base as the clash of different epistemological traditions – the formal and quantitative versus the qualitative and narrative-based – but that does not seem to be the key issue here. Rather, uneasiness about the evidence base comes from a sense that formal evidence is being used opportunistically and partially to substantiate a pre-determined policy position …

In particular, Needham and Glasby (2014) identify three key tensions over:

- *'Sequencing'* (with national policy often announcing the roll-out of new ways of working ahead of receiving the formal evidence).
- *'Interpretation'* (with different stakeholders disagreeing over what the emerging data means – see, for example, Slasberg et al, 2012a–b and Slasberg and Hatton, 2011 for debates around what the emerging data is telling us; see also Beresford, 2014a and Duffy, 2014 for discussions about the future of personalisation).
- Debates about what is *'relevant evidence'* in the first place.

Perhaps one example of the latter is a tendency in the personalisation literature to cite individual case studies as an illustration of the potential positives of this way of working (see Box 6.2 for examples). For advocates of personal budgets, these stories are a powerful way of illustrating the difference that personalisation can make, demonstrating in very real ways what can be achieved if traditional ways of thinking and of working are challenged and greater creativity is allowed to emerge. Above all, they start to show what can happen when people – whether service users and/or workers – start to genuinely believe that things can be different, push at the boundaries of what has previously been possible and build their confidence for the future by taking potentially small steps into the unknown. However, this use of individual stories has also attracted a significant backlash from those who feel that the case studies cited are unrepresentative of the people that use social care services more generally, that positive cases might have been 'cherry-picked' or that this is an attempt to 'sell' (Beresford, 2014a, p 160) a new way of working that may have significant negatives.

Box 6.2: The power of 'stories'

Charlie is a young man living in the countryside with a diagnosis of Paranoid Schizophrenia. After treatment for his mental health needs in hospital he returned to stay with his family but spent most of his time indoors. He felt unable to live in his own house, and had regular contact with mental health services. A personal budget enabled him to live at home with the support of personal assistants he and his family employed. Now he helps out on a local farm, his mental health has improved and he is living more independently.

Lynne was diagnosed with epilepsy after receiving a head injury and the impact of seizures on her everyday life was huge. Everyday tasks suddenly became hazardous to her. At her local Epilepsy Action branch she learned how Seizure Alert Dogs can warn epilepsy sufferers of imminent seizures. Lynne now uses her direct payment to fund the upkeep of her dog, Dougal.

David started his own business selling local produce at a market. His personal budget buys him support from a social enterprise that helps people with learning disabilities to establish their own micro-enterprises or small businesses.

(DH, 2010a, p 17)

While this is a broader issue than can be dealt with here, it is probably more than simply a discussion of whether personal budgets are a 'good' or a 'bad thing'. Elsewhere, we have argued that the current emphasis on 'evidence-based practice' in health and social care has become too dominated by formal research in general and by medical and quantitative research in particular (Glasby and Beresford, 2006; Glasby et al, 2007). Instead, Glasby and Beresford (2006) have called for a new notion of 'knowledge-based practice', combining different types of research, the practice wisdom of front-line staff and the lived experience of people who use services. Given that policy and front-line practice are nearly always ahead of the research evidence, this might represent a potentially exciting shift away from traditional 'evidence-based practice' and towards a form of 'practice-based evidence'. What is important, of course, is that individual stories include a range of positive and negative experiences, that effort is made to include 'seldom heard' voices and that individual case studies are considered alongside other forms of evidence and knowledge (including the findings of large national studies such as IBSEN). Stories, then, can be a powerful form of evidence and of communication – but part of their value may lie in the range of views sought, the rigour of the process and the willingness of everyone involved in these debates to explore the key issues in the round.

Aside from debates about the nature of the evidence base, a number of additional tensions have emerged over time as the adult social care system gains greater experience of implementing and working with personal budgets in practice. These are summarised in much greater detail in a companion volume (Needham and Glasby, 2014), and some of the potential pros and cons are explored in Chapters Seven and Eight of this book. However, key themes in these debates include some of the unresolved questions set out in Box 6.3, and it is important that everyone involved with adult social care has a view on these potential 'either-or' situations. For us, none of these potential dilemmas seems incapable of being solved, and many may be to do with the way personal budgets have been implemented, rather than the concept itself. Despite this, the fact remains that both supporters and critics of the personalisation agenda have strong views on these issues, and those working in adult social care will have to find ways of resolving such potential tensions in their own practice and local context to the best of their ability (see the reflective exercises at the end of this chapter for further details).

In spite of all the dilemmas listed in Box 6.3, our belief is that there are two particular tensions that remain unresolved and that are potentially even more significant than the ones raised above:

1. Personal budgets were developed by people committed to greater citizenship – more of a civil rights movement than a traditional social care policy. Yet, the current financial context is such that the potential positives of personal budgets could be almost entirely undermined by the broader austerity agenda in public services (see, O'Hara, 2014, for examples of the impact of recent cuts; see also Pearson et al, 2014, ch 5 for a discussion of personalisation in an era of austerity). This point has been made particularly forcefully by Simon Duffy, one of the key figures in the development of personal budgets, who has accused the Coalition government of 2010–15 of waging an unprecedented campaign against the rights of disabled people with dramatic cuts in social care, benefits and housing (Duffy, 2013 – see also Duffy, 2012a for his analysis of 'is personalisation dead?'). This is strong stuff, but it certainly seems counter-productive to be offering a policy badged as promoting choice and control over social care support at the same time as a series of funding cuts that may make meaningful choice and control much harder in the other parts of people's lives. In response, supporters of personal budgets will need to reflect on to what extent they believe personalisation can really deliver in the current context,

while critics could ask themselves whether some of their critique is more to do with the broader financial context than with personal budgets per se.

Box 6.3: Key questions about the impact of personal budgets

From the beginning, personalisation has been the subject of significant debate and controversy. Approaching the issues from different standpoints and perspectives, different commentators have seen personalisation either as a radical revolution in which services are transformed and power shifted dramatically in favour of people using services or an attempt to roll back the boundaries of the welfare state, undermine public sector services and pass off state responsibilities onto people already in need. As the implications of personalisation have started to become clearer over time, key questions have included:

- Is personalisation transferring risk and responsibility from the state to the individual – or is it promoting more of a partnership of equals in which risk is shared in a positive way by the individual and the system together?
- Is personalisation connecting people more fully with their family, friends and communities – or is it closing down collective spaces such as day centres and isolating people in their homes?
- Can personalisation work equally well for all types of people using services – and in particular for older people?
- Will personalisation free people up to choose what sort of relationship they want with their friends and families – or will it place an unacceptable burden on unpaid women carers?
- How can the positive approaches to risk inherent in personalisation be reconciled with safeguarding?
- Will personalisation deepen inequalities between people using social care services – or more fully tailor responses to individual need so that outcomes are more equal?
- Is personalisation de-professionalising social workers and depressing terms and conditions for the broader social care workforce – or will it lead to a return to the values of community social work and to better relationships between care workers and their employers?
- Is personalisation adding to bureaucracy and legal ambiguity – or is it simplifying people's entitlement to resources?
- Is personalisation a concept that could revolutionise other areas of the welfare state – or is it being stretched into other sectors (such as health) on the basis of a weak evidence base?

Depending on where you sit, personalisation is either the best thing since sliced bread or the end of the welfare state as we know it – and it's often hard to find much common ground between these two opposing stances. Only half in jest has all this been dubbed a 'Marmite' issue – with personalisation rapidly emerging as something that people either love or hate.

(Needham and Glasby, 2014, pp 4–5)

2. Although we firmly believe that personal budgets have the potential to achieve positive outcomes, there is always a risk that they will be implemented badly (or for motives other than those of the original designers of this way of working). Again, this risk has been highlighted by Simon Duffy, who argues passionately that any system has a series of self-defence mechanisms against external challenge and can easily appropriate the language of reform while quietly watering things down and maintaining the status quo. For him, we now have a form of 'zombie personalisation' (Duffy, 2014, p 178) in too many areas of the country: that looks nearly like the real thing, but is really just a pale imitation. Although some areas have remained committed to the underlying principles of personalisation (Barnsley is named as a good-practice example), Duffy (2012a) identifies a series of implementation problems, including:

- 'The rationing process (known as the RAS) is often too bureaucratic and too complex and yet ambiguous
- The RAS is also being used to make cuts in ways that seem unreasonable and are possibly illegal
- The planning process has become more burdensome, with disabled people and families forced to get their own plans through a panel of managers
- Expensive monitoring systems take away real flexibility and damage independence
- Little effort has been made to redesign systems to make them more workable for people or social workers
- Some people are assigned budgets, but lack the means to control them.'

As Duffy (2012a) concludes: 'at times it is hard to stay positive. Much has been achieved, but so much more could be achieved' – see also Duffy (2012b) for an 'apology' in response to the tendency for some areas to develop overly complex resource allocation systems and to the 'industry' that has grown up around support planning). Certainly, there seem to be some fairly spurious practices at work in some local localities, with some people allegedly receiving a personal budget apparently unaware that they are, or not knowing what is available to spend. While there is often a mismatch between what councils feel they are doing and how people receiving services perceive it, we would argue that if someone doesn't know they have a personal budget, then they really don't have one (whatever exists on paper). As with direct payments, a personal budget is only a mechanism, and its impact will depend on how individual workers and local areas choose to use this mechanism. For Duffy (2012b), part of the way forward is therefore to:

- 'Avoid solving false problems, problems that are not real but are just symptoms of a flawed system
- Keep innovating, finding simpler and more respectful solutions to real problems
- Challenge injustice, don't accept unfair cuts or damaging policies
- Build community, share our ideas and be prepared to listen, learn and change.'

The experience of different user groups and different areas of the country

As personal budgets have grown in number and become more mainstream, there is evidence to suggest that different areas of the country are implementing the personalisation agenda in different ways. In England, the annual ADASS (2014) personalisation survey found that 81% of all people receiving community-based services were supported by personal budgets or direct payments, albeit there were 'wide regional variations in delivery: perhaps too wide yet to be confident that these policies are embedded' (p 4). Only a very small proportion of people receiving a personal budget (4%) did so via an individual service fund, and this potential mechanism seems to be significantly under-utilised to date.

With greater opposition to perceived market-based reforms, Scotland has adopted a slightly different approach (see Pearson et al, 2014 for a summary), with specific legislation (the Social Care (Self-Directed Support) Act 2013) and a series of options as to how people with social care needs exercise choice and control over their support (see also Chapter Three). As the Scottish Government's Self-Directed Support website (www.selfdirectedsupportscotland.org.uk/) explains:

> Self-directed support includes a range of options to ensure everyone can exercise choice and control:
>
> - a Direct Payment (a cash payment);
> - funding allocated to a provider of your choice (sometimes called an individual service fund, where the council holds the budget but the person is in charge of how it is spent);
> - the council can arrange a service for you; or
> - you can choose a mix of these options for different types of support.

In Wales, there remain official concerns that personal budgets could undermine existing public services (see, for example, Lombard, 2009). Organisations such as the Welsh Alliance for Citizen Directed Services (formerly In Control Cymru) are seeking to develop other ways of achieving greater self-direction (see http://wacds.org.uk). In Northern Ireland, numbers have been very low, albeit there is an aspiration to mainstream personal budgets (arguably from a low base). As part of a draft equality impact assessment, Northern Ireland's Health and Social Care Board has stated (2015, p 14):

> As part of the Transforming Your Care programme of change, this project sets out to mainstream Self Directed Support as a realistic alternative to traditional services, for those individuals with eligible needs. By 31st March 2018 it is envisaged that 1 in 3 eligible Service Users will avail of Self Directed Support across all Trusts.

In many ways, this seems similar to the initial expansion of direct payments (see Chapters Three and Four), with different histories and political traditions in different areas of the country arguably influencing local attitudes and approaches. As was also the case with direct payments, there is emerging evidence to suggest that different user groups may be experiencing personal budgets in different ways (although there is always a risk, in making such statements, of resorting to generalisations about whole groups of people). This is not explored in detail here, as many of the themes here are similar to the earlier experience of direct payments in Chapter Four. However, Box 6.4 summarises some potentially familiar themes around the experiences of groups such as older people and people with mental health problems (see also Newbronner et al, 2011). In trying to make sense of these findings, we would argue that:

1. Despite differential experiences, it still seems as if personal budgets can produce potential benefits for a range of different groups. For us, there is no evidence to suggest that 'personal budgets can't work for older people' (or for another group). While older people to date might have different experiences of personal budgets, there are still potential positives for which to strive. Although we would not put it as strongly as this, some might even argue that saying 'personal budgets can't work for older people' is almost a form of ageism in itself – and is arguably a statement to be challenged.

2. Having said this, the history and culture of different user group settings is such that personal budgets may play out differently for different people – and we may need to work harder in some settings. As with the direct payments literature (and simplified above), a particular focus has often been on the experiences of older people, with fears that older people's care is so under-funded that only very basic care tasks can be undertaken. Put another way, the level of funding might be such that there is no real scope for innovation and creativity, irrespective of whether someone has a personal budget or not. For us, this is the result of broader inequities in the way services are organised, not the fault of personal budgets (indeed it is even arguable that the advent of personal budgets might help to make these issues more transparent and therefore give greater scope for them to be challenged). However, the fact remains that some workers (and older people's services are probably a good example) may need to be particularly dogged and innovative if personal budgets are to be genuinely embedded in everyday services.

The spread to other sectors

The spread of personal budgets has been rapid in adult social care, and it has also started to extend into other service settings. As set out in Chapter Five, the initial Department of Health pilots sought to test not the In Control 'personal budget' (adult social care only), but a broader 'individual budget' (a more integrated

> ## Box 6.4: The experience of different user groups
>
> Despite significant positives for younger age groups, early research suggested that older people might not benefit to the same extent (see, for example, Glendinning et al, 2008; Woolham and Benton, 2012). This has led to a series of reviews, new research, case studies and good practice guidance (see, for example, DH, 2010b; Alzheimer's Society, 2011; Mental Health Foundation, 2011; Baxter et al, 2013; Routledge and Carr, 2013; Woolham, 2013; Zamfir, 2013; Ellis Paine et al, 2014; Routledge et al, 2015), many suggesting that personal budgets can have a positive impact for older people – but that there are a series of additional barriers to overcome in this setting.
>
> In mental health services, concerns about levels of take-up of personal budgets led to a systematic review of the evidence (Webber et al, 2014 – see also Larsen et al, 2013 and NHS Confederation, 2015 for further discussion). As Webber et al (2014, p 153) conclude:
>
>> To the best of our knowledge, this is the only systematic review of the international literature on the effectiveness of personal budgets for people with mental health problems. It has found generally positive outcomes for mental health service users in terms of choice and control, impact on quality of life, service use, and cost-effectiveness. However, methodological limitations make these findings rather unreliable and insufficient to inform policy and practice. There is a need for large high quality experimental studies in this key policy area to inform personal budget policy and practice with people with mental health problems.

funding pot with scope to include funds from sources such as social care, the Independent Living Fund, Access to Work, and funds for aids and adaptations). While some saw this as an ambitious extension of the initial concept, others felt that there was a real risk of 'running before we could walk' and that policy would have been better to concentrate initially on adult social care. Indeed, the risk was even that the pilots would fail – not because personal budgets do not work but because of an arguably slightly naïve attempt to join up funding streams that are very difficult to combine. Certainly, these fears seemed to be backed up by IBSEN, which identified positive outcomes for personal budgets but very little progress (not to mention significant frustration) around the complexity of seeking to integrate other sources of funding:

> Support for the integration or alignment of most funding streams was, in principle, positive … However, the majority of IB [individual budget] and funding stream leads whom we interviewed were disappointed at the slow progress with the integration of other funding streams despite significant local investment in understanding how the different funding streams operated and how integration might be achieved … IB lead officers reported their frustration that integration had been limited by a perceived lack of commitment and/or over

cautiousness at national level ... Eligibility criteria for adult social care did not fully overlap with that for the other funding streams; assessment processes and review arrangements had only been integrated or aligned (in some sites) for [two of the various funding streams]; and most IB lead officers reported little, if any, flexibility in how monies for non-social care funding streams could be used by an IB holder. Some IB lead officers argued that the limited coverage and short-term nature of the IB Pilot Projects may have inhibited central government's willingness to amend the legal and governance restrictions that inhibited closer integration at local levels. (Glendinning et al, 2008, pp 114 and 139)

Despite these initial findings, attempts to explore the concept of personal budgets have continued in a range of different setting (see Box 6.5). Although it is beyond the immediate scope of this book, the Health Services Management Centre and the Centre for Welfare Reform have produced a series of policy papers on the implications of personalisation for health care, for disabled children, for community development, for criminal justice and for the tax and benefits system (Alakeson, 2010b; Murray, 2010; Gillespie with Hughes, 2010; Hyde, 2010; Duffy, 2010). As outlined above, personal budgets represent not just a change to the social care system but, potentially, a shift in the relationship between the state and the individual. In a period of demographic pressures, advances in medicine and technology, changes in family structures and rising public expectations, such a shift seems to offer a potential way forward for welfare services more generally. As the think-tank Demos has argued, possible areas where such an approach might work could include job search and employment, drug user and offender rehabilitation, young people not in education, employment or training, and supporting families at risk (Leadbeater et al, 2008). Similarly, Duffy (2008) has suggested that the principles of self-directed support could be applied in areas such as community development, services for people dependent on drugs or alcohol, education, employment and housing. Viewed from this angle, personal budgets – although originating in social care – could form a significant part of future welfare reform.

Of all the areas where personal budgets could be extended, one of the most prominent seems to be health care – not least because of the scale of the NHS, its popularity with the public and the controversies that can arise if changes are seen to represent a degree of 'privatisation' (although see Powell, 2015; Powell and Miller, 2014 for a more detailed critique of what privatisation might actually mean in an NHS context). Despite ongoing emphasis on joint working between health and social care, both direct payments and personal budgets were actively promoted in social care at the same time (until recently) as they were being actively ruled out in health care (DH, 2006, p 85). While an extension of direct payments to some forms of health care has periodically been suggested (see, for example, Glendinning et al, 2000a–c; Glasby and Hasler, 2004; Glasby and Duffy, 2007), it was not until 2007–08 that the momentum for change seemed to gather pace

Box 6.5: Extending to other settings

Initial individual budget pilots sought to combine funding from adult social care, the Independent Living Fund, Access to Work and various equipment and housing-related funds. Local sites struggled to integrate these different funding pots (which would arguably need much more fundamental national action to be successful). Despite this, subsequent 'Right to Control trailblazers' (under the Welfare Reform Act 2009) sought to do something very similar – bringing together funding from Access to Work, adult social care, the Disabled Facilities Grant, the Independent Living Fund, Supporting People and Work Choice in seven pilot sites. The evaluation concluded that '[we] did not find any evidence of the Right to Control having a significant positive impact on customers ... The primary potential explanations for this are that many customers were not following the intended Right to Control customer journey and that provider markets were not yet sufficiently developed to offer meaningful choice. Trailblazers were working to overcome these issues but success depended on a considerable culture change among staff, customers and providers, which could not be fully realised within the relatively short timeframe of the pilot' (Tu et al, 2013, p 3).

While the language in IBSEN and the Right to Control evaluation has to be neutral, a lay reader might read between the lines to conclude that both these attempts at high-profile national initiatives/local pilots struggled to be meaningful – in strong contrast to the positives achieved more bottom-up via the In Control personal budget pilots. This is not to say that integrating different funding sources cannot work – in many ways it makes perfect sense and, in future, it may become the norm. However, some would argue that national policy does not have a good track record of taking bottom-up initiatives, rolling out effectively and staying true to their underlying principles. As Moran et al (2011, p 240) argue:

> [These initiatives] exemplify a profound failure of joined-up government. Indeed, rather than moving towards greater flexibility and integration of resource streams, the subsequent proliferation of individual-budget type initiatives carries the imprint of individual departmental resource and ministerial silos.

Although personal budgets developed initially in adult social care, there have been a series of attempts to develop similar approaches in children's services – whether this is In Control's 'Children's Programme' (www.in-control.org.ukwhat-we-do/children-and-young-people.aspx), national 'budget-holding lead professional' pilots (Walker et al, 2009), for children with special educational needs (Prabhakar et al, 2011; Department for Education, 2012; see also Murray, 2010 for a broader discussion), or in adoption services (Samuel, 2013).

Given the growing focus on the relationship between health and social care, there have been growing calls over time to develop more personalised approaches within the NHS (see below for further discussion of personal health budgets).

There have also been additional pilots seeking to develop personal budgets/more personalised approaches in services for rough sleepers (Hough and Rice, 2010; Blackender and Prestidge, 2014) and in terms of the resettlement of offenders leaving prison (Moore and Nicol, 2009; Dickie, 2013).

(see Harding, 2005; Alakeson, 2007, 2010b; Conservative Party, 2007; Le Grand, 2007; Milburn, 2007; Brown, 2008; Darzi, 2008; Glasby, 2008; Glendinning et al, 2008; Leadbeater et al, 2008). After significant debate, New Labour introduced a series of personal health budget pilots (with direct payments an active option for some sites under the Health Act 2009). The subsequent evaluation found that personal health budgets improve quality of life and are cost-effective (Forder et al, 2012; www.phbe.org.uk; see Slasberg et al, 2014 for an opposing view). There has since been an announcement that personal health budgets will be extended to people receiving NHS continuing health care (DH, 2011a), significant work to explore the implications for mental health services (Alakeson and Perkins, 2012; NHS Confederation, 2015 – see Welch et al, 2013 for discussion of the implications for substance misuse services) and ongoing attempts to implement in settings such as services for people with long-term conditions (see Alakeson, 2014 for an introductory guide to personal health budgets). More recently, the *NHS Mandate* sets out an expectation that people with long-term conditions (including people with mental health problems) who could benefit should have the choice of a personal health budget (DH, 2014b), while NHS England (2014) has signalled its intention to deliver personal budgets made up of more integrated health and social care funding (which it describes as 'integrated personal commissioning').

As a result of all this, personal budgets are important not just in their own right, but also for their potential impact across a range of services. Elsewhere, personal budgets have been characterised as a form of 'Conditional Resource Enhancement' (CRE), with Waters and Duffy (2007) suggesting that it is possible for governments to seek to meet the needs of their citizens via a combination of five different approaches (see Figure 6.1):

Figure 6.1: Five different strategies for improved well-being

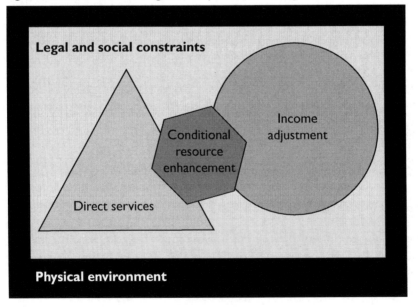

- *Create legal and social structures*: the legal system can impose obligations on people to act fairly and can punish those who might act in ways that damage well-being (e.g. disability discrimination legislation aims to protect disabled people from unfair treatment).
- *Adjust income*: the tax and benefit system enables government to alter the resources people can control directly and the incentives under which they operate (e.g. social security payments to disabled people or tax credits to ease transition back to work for people who are unemployed).
- *Direct service*: the government provides, directly or indirectly, a range of health, educational or other services that people either must or can use, subject to whatever criteria govern eligibility to that service.
- *Adapt physical environment*: the government can change the structure of the environment within which the person operates (e.g. increasingly buildings are designed so as to enable people who use wheelchairs full physical access).
- *Conditional Resource Enhancement*: the government can also target resources towards those individuals who are eligible, but with specific conditions attached (e.g. personal budgets).

Viewed from this angle, the advent of personal budgets might be seen as arising as the government finds that funding, currently committed to direct services, is better managed by people themselves. Shifting resources into the form of a CRE could therefore be a way of improving the management of those resources, while still achieving the same social objectives. While these ideas are complex and are still developing, this new concept of a CRE might involve:

- *Autonomy*: the CRE must be under the control of the individual or of someone who can properly represent their interests.
- *Flexibility*: the CRE must be able to be put to different uses by the person – it cannot be so inflexible that it cannot be shaped by the person.
- *Targeting*: the person receiving the CRE must be eligible in some way for receiving the CRE.
- *Support*: the person receiving the CRE may get some form of support, information or advice.
- *Conditionality*: there must be some conditions, the breach of which would enable the CRE to be constrained, withdrawn or managed in some different way.

While this is discussed in more detail elsewhere (Waters and Duffy, 2007), a personal budget seems to be a particularly pure and strong form of CRE. Whereas other potential CREs (for example, wheelchair vouchers or Local Housing Allowance) tend to place heavy restrictions on *how* the CRE can be used, personal budgets focus on the purpose of the CRE and upon the *outcomes* that it is meant to achieve. This seems a particularly helpful approach if we are to assume that the individual citizen is best placed to decide how their needs should be met and that historical services are not necessarily the best guide as to what will be appropriate in the future. In addition, it is interesting to note that some previous CREs (for example, the notorious Individual Learning Account scheme) have been dogged by allegations of misuse, fraud and theft. In contrast, both direct payments and personal budgets (to date) seem to have been remarkably free of such abuse. While it is too early to know, one possible lesson here is that approaches that place resources under the control of those with the biggest vested interest in spending them effectively may be the safest way of managing resources.

Aside from being of intellectual interest, this discussion is helpful in so far as it enables us to explore possible approaches to future welfare reform. It is probably still too early to be clear, but at least three possibilities seem to exist.

- Personal budgets may be only a transitional measure, allowing resources to shift from the state to the individual without completely disrupting social expectations about the state's duty to guarantee welfare for people who are perceived to be entitled to support by the general public. On this account, the CRE is a transitional state, and personal budgets may well become a form of income adjustment over time.
- It may be that the dynamic interaction or co-production now possible between professionals and the users of personal budgets is the optimal state for improving well-being and personal outcomes for the people who currently use social care. On this account, the CRE is the end-state and the extension of personal budgets will signify a significant new phase in the development of the welfare state.
- Against this, it is also possible that the development of personal budgets may lead to attempts to shift more private income or benefits into the framework of the CRE (although this is not advocated by the current authors). This is a very different strategic direction, reducing the level of resources over which the individual has autonomous control. For example, a possible option for the reform of English long-term care has sometimes included the notion of a 'partnership model' (Wanless, 2006) in which the state guarantees to pay a certain proportion of the cost of such support and the individual makes up the difference (either via personal savings/income or via the social security system for those on low incomes). In future, it would be perfectly possible for such a model to be implemented via a CRE. Similarly, there might be scope to shift some social security payments (such as current disability benefits) into the CRE framework. Thus, while personal budgets have been developed in the context of trying to shift control away from direct services and towards the individual, this is not the only possible direction – it is also possible to use CREs to make resources that were clearly under the control of the individual more conditional.

SUMMARY

Since the publication of the IBSEN evaluation in 2008, our knowledge of what works and our experience of working with personal budgets in practice have both continued to grow. Although there have been significant positives, there have also been a number of tensions as an initially small-scale innovation has become national policy and has been rolled out everywhere at pace and scale. In such circumstances, it is probably unsurprising that the spread of personal budgets has been different in different parts of the country and in different user group settings – or that different views have developed about the strengths and limitations of this way of working. Despite this – and in spite of heated views for and against – everyone receiving adult social care should do so via a personal budget (with direct payments as the default option). There have also been a series of potentially significant extensions to other sectors (especially to health care), and interest remains in exploring scope for personalisation to become a more general principle of broader welfare services. However, Simon Duffy's claim that too many parts of the country are introducing 'zombie personalisation' remains a serious one – and all of us have a responsibility to reflect whether this is true of us, our practice, our local services and the social care system more generally. Compared to the second edition of this book, the current chapter is less optimistic, more mixed and perhaps better at identifying questions and dilemmas than it is at giving answers – but the fact remains that personal budgets are still 'the only game in town'.

IMPLICATIONS FOR POLICY AND PRACTICE

- For all the debates in this chapter, personal budgets seem to have the potential to achieve significant benefits. While the initial enthusiasm of the late 2000s has perhaps given way to a more cautious response, the evidence seems clear that (implemented well) personal budgets can make a positive difference to people's lives.
- This is arguably true for all user groups, but we may need to work harder and to work differently in some settings. This might be more to do with the history and culture of different settings than it is to do with personal budgets per se.
- As personal budgets have been rolled out, a number of tensions and quite significantly different viewpoints have emerged. Some of these may be more to do with the way in which personal budgets have been implemented rather than inherent in the concept – but this is contested.
- For workers, there is no choice but to implement national policy – but there remains a choice as to how well personal budgets are implemented locally and around how individual practitioners try to maximise the opportunities and minimise the limitations.
- In terms of national policy, there is a challenge as to how the underlying value base of personal budgets can be maintained as they become part mainstream policy, especially in a challenging policy and financial context. There may also be an in-built tendency for existing systems to resist innovation, quietly finding ways of recreating themselves under the guise of new language.

RECOMMENDED READING AND USEFUL WEBSITES

Since our second edition, there is now much more material exploring the impact of personal budgets, lessons learnt from working with them in practice and resources for policy makers, practitioners and people using services.

In terms of numbers and spread, the national ADASS personalisation survey sets out annual data (in England) for some 132 (87%) councils, looking at overall numbers, geographical spread and expenditure, as well as qualitative assessments around topics such as workforce, assessment processes, information and advice, support planning and market facilitation (see, for example, ADASS, 2014). Data for other parts of the UK is typically harder to extract but updates and future plans can usually be found in the latest strategy documents from the relevant national Parliament/Assembly.

In terms of emerging good practice and accessible guidance/resources, TLAP is a national partnership of more than 50 organisations seeking to transform services through personalisation. Its website includes lots of helpful, practical material, as well as case studies, stories and practical lessons learned locally (see www.thinklocalactpersonal.org.uk). As an example, its 2011 publication on *Taking Stock, Moving Forward* provides a snapshot of the emerging evidence at that time, makes recommendations for future policy and practice and provides further resources (TLAP, 2011c).

From a more academic perspective, the work of Catherine Needham explores the spread of personalisation to other sectors – and tries to do this by understanding the nature and the rationale behind these extensions, rather than necessarily commenting on whether or not this is a good thing (see, for example, Needham, 2010, 2011).

For those interested in personal health budgets, Vidhya Alakeson has produced research into the US experience of similar approaches, promoted this way of working in the UK and produced practical guidance and advice for NHS colleagues wanting to understand and implement personal health budgets (see Alakeson, 2007, 2010a, 2010b, 2014).

For a summary of some of the debates between supporters and critics of personalisation, see Needham and Glasby's (2014) edited collection, *Debates in Personalisation* (also published by The Policy Press). With contributions from different stakeholders involved in implementing and exploring the impact of personal budgets, this book tries to highlight some of the very different (and often opposing) views which exist in a contested area of policy and practice. The final chapters by Peter Beresford and by Simon Duffy are particularly useful summaries of different viewpoints, and the book is designed to be provocative, critical and, hopefully, helpful. Other contributions by Slasberg et al (2012a–b) and by Beresford (2011/12) provide a critique of personal budgets, while Zarb (2013) describes personalisation as a form of 'independent living lite.'

REFLECTIVE EXERCISES

1. Supporters and critics of personal budgets alike have much to say – but what in your personal experience is the impact of personal budgets (whether you have used services, worked in them and/or formed a view from the material in this book)? If you had to choose, would you want a personal budget (for you or for a family member/friend) and what pros and cons might this have, from your point of view?

2. Based on the experience of adult social care, do personal budgets have a potential contribution to make in other sectors of the welfare state? If so, which ones – and what might be the issues involved in introducing this way of working in these settings? Is there anything you can do to use your knowledge of personal budgets to help colleagues in other sectors learn from the experience in social care?

3. Reflecting on the 'either-or' questions in Box 6.3, where would you position yourself on this spectrum of options/interpretations? For each bullet point, ask yourself: what do I think personal budgets are achieving here, and what could I do to build on the potential positives and limit the possible negatives?

SEVEN

The advantages of direct payments and personal budgets

This chapter explores the impact of direct payments and personal budgets in terms of:
- choice and control;
- morale and well-being;
- positive changes in people's lives;
- use of resources.

Over time, many of the advocates and critics of both direct payments and personal budgets have set out strong views (ourselves included) – but with a lot of debate taking place in the early days of new approaches, ahead of more detailed experience of working with new concepts in practice and ahead of the formal research evidence. This has been exacerbated by the pace of national policy, with new ways of working often rolled out ahead of the evidence base. To some extent this is inevitable – policy and practice are always ahead of the formal research, and it is sometimes necessary to make changes to systems that do not seem to be working in order to learn by doing and reflecting. However, the fact remains that there is significant merit in returning to the underlying research in order to get a better understanding of potential advantages (this chapter) and limitations (Chapter Eight), before forming a view as to next steps and implications (see the Conclusion to this book). Given that the literature is now expanding rapidly, this chapter and Chapter Eight both try to highlight some key issues and to give a flavour of the evidence, without claiming to be exhaustive. To give a sense of the way in which research has developed over time, we tend to focus in detail on some of the early findings as new ways of working were being introduced, and then on the extent to which initial aspirations have been backed up in practice by more recent evaluation.

Choice and control

In the early 1990s, research into the ILF revealed that making cash payments directly to service users gave a sense of control and choice that could not be achieved via statutory services (Kestenbaum, 1993a–b; Lakey, 1994; see also Chapter Two). While respondents found directly provided services to be inflexible, costly and severely limited in terms of the availability and level of service on offer, they valued the freedom that ILF payments provided. Receiving money with which to employ their own care assistants enabled them to choose staff who they felt had the right strengths and skills. The disabled person could also employ someone of a particular gender and could select carers who spoke the same language as they did. Above all, ILF recipients valued being able to hire staff with whom they felt able to develop a good relationship, choosing people with the right personality to make the care package work. As a result, the disabled people were able to establish and maintain longer-lasting relationships with their staff and enjoyed greater continuity of personnel. At the same time, they were also able to create flexible support arrangements to meet often-fluctuating needs. Throughout a number of research studies, respondents repeatedly emphasised the control that ILF payments gave them and the self-respect that they felt as a result of their status as an employer. Rather than being dependent on others to determine and meet their care needs, the disabled people themselves could determine what Kestenbaum (1993b, p 38) describes as 'the what, how, who and when of care arrangements'.

In 1993, respondents in Morris's study of disabled people's experiences of community care emphasised the many advantages that employing PAs could bring:

> "I'm a husband, a father and a breadwinner. And ten years ago I was in an institution where I couldn't even decide when I would go to the toilet."

> "It means that I can get up in the morning when I want to, and lead the kind of life that I want to ... To not be reliant on my family and friends ... to keep all that separate [so that] to them I'm me rather than someone who needs help."

> "It means exercising choice and control, having the right to choose who gets me up and who puts me to bed."

> "I'm living on my own, living in the way I like. I can come and go as I like."

> "I employ people ..., which allows me to have the life style that I choose."

> (Quoted in Morris, 1993a, pp 125–6)

In 1994, similar findings emerged from Zarb and Nadash's study for BCODP. For many respondents, indirect/direct payments were crucial in enabling recipients to control the times when support was provided, who was employed, what sort of assistance was provided and how it was provided, thereby enhancing quality of life and personal dignity. Overall, the most important aspect of a payments scheme was found to be having choice and control over one's own support arrangements. This in turn led to more reliable and flexible services that enabled needs to be more fully met.

Following the Community Care (Direct Payments) Act 1996, further research and practical experience has emphasised the centrality of choice and control (see, for example, Hasler et al, 1999; Dawson, 2000; Leece, 2000; Vasey, 2000; Witcher et al, 2000; CSCI, 2004; Stainton and Boyce, 2004). As one participant in a service user-controlled review of direct payments in Wiltshire suggested:

> "There are times when I just put my head in my hands and wonder why on earth I am putting myself through all the hassle of employing people when I could theoretically receive an equivalent service ... Yet I then remember starting out on a service and know that I could never go back to that, although at the time I thought the service was good. The quality and flexibility I now have is because I have an individually designed package to suit not just myself but also my family and lifestyle and it is worth every second of any stress." (Quoted in Carmichael and Brown, 2002, p 800)

With the advent of personal budgets, both research and practice have continued to stress the importance of choice and control. Thus, Poll et al's (2006) evaluation of the first six In Control case study sites found that the number of people satisfied with the amount of control they had over their lives increased from 42% to 97% as a result of receiving a personal budget (p 41). This was confirmed in 2008, when monitoring suggested that 72% of participants reported improvements in choice and control, with 27% reporting no change and only 1% saying that things had got worse since starting self-directed support (Hatton et al, 2008, p 20). By 2014, the third national personal budget survey found that 70% of people felt that personal budgets had led to a positive impact in terms of being in control of their life (Waters and Hatton, 2014). However, as suggested in Chapter Eight, concerns remain that initial gains around greater choice and control can be lost if personal budgets are implemented badly, if new systems are overly bureaucratic and/or if new ways of working are used as a smokescreen for austerity (see also Duffy, 2012a, 2012b, 2014 for discussion of the fragility of recent gains and the scope for promising innovations to be resisted, co-opted and watered down).

Morale and well-being

For direct payment and personal budget recipients, feeling in control of their own lives seems to have important implications for health and well-being. There is a large literature in the field of psychology to suggest that control is essential to well-being and an important element in shaping people's lives and their susceptibility to stress. Often, psychologists distinguish between people who have an internal or an external 'locus of control'. Whereas 'internals' feel in control of what happens to them and that they have the power to influence their lives, 'externals' tend to believe that they have little control over what happens to them, since this is the result of outside factors beyond their command (Thompson et al, 1994, pp 54–5). This can be crucial, since research suggests that 'internals' are more successful than 'externals' in the workplace in terms of pay, promotion and job satisfaction, and that they are better able to cope with stress (Andrisani and Nestel, 1976). This has been supported by Kobasa (1979), who suggests that people with a greater sense of control over what happens to them will remain healthier than those who feel powerless in the face of external forces. Another key contribution has been made by Seligman (1975), who believes that 'externals' are more likely to experience 'learned helplessness' (where people who constantly find that they have little power to influence their own destiny lose motivation and give up trying).

With regard to social care, evidence is beginning to emerge that the increased sense of control that receiving direct payments and personal budgets entails can enhance well-being and morale. Certainly, this was one of the early findings to emerge from research into the ILF, which suggested that receiving cash payments enabled some disabled people to remain in the community rather than enter hospital or residential care (Kestenbaum, 1993b). For one service user, Mr R, ILF payments gave him the confidence to do other things, safe in the knowledge that the physical side of his care was under control and that his support arrangements were keeping pressure sores at bay (Kestenbaum, 1993b, p 39). As the government was considering the potential of direct payments in the mid-1990s, John Evans, then chair of BCODP's Independent Living Committee, was clear that direct payments would have a direct effect on people's quality of life:

> Direct payments allow disabled people to be less dependent, to have real choices about how we live our lives … They have a real impact on quality of life – on health, wellbeing, psychological development, and relationships with others. (Quoted in George, 1994, p 14)

After the introduction of direct payments in 1996/97, research conducted by the PSI/NCIL suggested that replacing directly provided services with cash payments may not only be more cost-efficient, but might also bring a range of additional social and economic benefits:

> Savings may come from a reduction in demand for acute and/or long-term health care on the basis that full independence may well be associated with higher levels of quality of life and the associated benefits in terms of general well-being. (Zarb, 1998, pp 8–9)

Improved mental and physical health was also a key outcome for disabled people during research into direct payments and the health and social care divide (Glendinning et al, 2000a, 2000c). For many direct payment recipients, enhanced choice and control increased their self-confidence, morale and emotional and psychological health in a range of areas. For some respondents, the depth of their relationship with their PA was a crucial source of support and helped to prevent feelings of isolation. For others, the quality of care that they were able to arrange for themselves had a knock-on effect on their attitude to their impairments and symptoms. This was particularly the case for people with mental health problems, who felt that direct payments gave them the confidence and support they needed to recover from their illness. In the same way, Stainton and Boyce (2004) found that direct payments can bring significant psychological benefits, increasing people's confidence, making them feel more optimistic about their lives and motivating them to explore new avenues (p 451):

> "It's built up my self-esteem, given me a lot more confidence, made me feel I'm part of the real world, not just a drag on it physically and financially ... I feel now my horizons are limitless."

> "I have got my life back ... I have got choice. I can do things ... No such word as can't or no or you shouldn't."

With the advent of personal budgets, the impact on health and well-being appears to be even more pronounced. In one sense, this is to be expected from the international evidence, with a summary of US research (Alakeson, 2007) suggesting that outcomes could well improve under self-directed support, with self-direction believed to promote prevention and early intervention to a greater extent than traditional services (which focus more on intervening after a crisis). More recently, the national personal budgets survey suggests positive impacts in terms of mental health, feeling safe, family relationships, friendships and self-esteem (Waters and Hatton, 2014), while IBSEN and the national evaluation of personal health budgets found evidence of people feeling their aspirations had changed, that people felt they were leading a fuller life and that psychological well-being had improved (Glendinning et al, 2008; Forder et al, 2012). As personal budgets extend further into the NHS, there may be even greater scope for positive outcomes in future in this regard.

Outcomes and positive change

While choice and control are important ends in themselves, the practical upshot seems to be the increased ability for people to make changes in their lives and to achieve outcomes that are meaningful to them. In one sense, this is a theme that runs throughout this book, and almost all of the case studies and research findings cited in other chapters illustrate the potential of direct payments and personal budgets to transform people's lives. In many ways, both direct payments and personal budgets seem to operate very much like pebbles thrown into a pond, with ripples that spread out much further than their initial impact (both in terms of the life of the individual and throughout the social care system more generally). Certainly, this was one of the findings from Stainton and Boyce's (2004) review of direct payments in two Welsh local authorities, with the authors noting how direct payments had 'permeated aspects of the lives of many users well beyond the direct influence of their care package' (p 449). Interestingly, the greater choice and control experienced by direct payment recipients in this study was also felt to help them live life-styles less constrained by externally imposed routines, and a number of participants in the study were engaged in voluntary work, were attending vocational courses or were using personal assistance when at work. Given the national emphasis that is now being placed on lifelong learning, on voluntary work and on supporting disabled people to engage in paid employment, the potential impact of direct payments in this area seems worthy of further exploration.

In addition, the findings of early In Control evaluations illustrate the way in which self-directed support can enable people to make desired changes to their lives and achieve a range of outcomes that matter to them. Thus, as Chapter Five demonstrated, many early personal budget holders were able to design support that enabled them to reduce their use of institutional forms of service provision, make more use of community supports and play a greater role in their communities – all within a relatively short period of time and for either the same or less money than their original support package (see Box 7.1 for further examples). However, behind these findings there seems to be a more fundamental point about the nature of direct payments and personal budgets. While previous approaches have often been very service-led (essentially slotting people into pre-existing and pre-purchased services), direct payments and personal budgets have the potential to focus on assessed needs, allowing individuals and their networks to be more creative in terms of how they go about meeting these needs (and to do so in a way that achieves outcomes that make sense to the individual in the context of their own life, community and aspirations). Viewed from this angle, direct payments and personal budgets are less about money changing hands than they are about freeing people up to make much better and more meaningful decisions about meeting needs. As one individual budget holder in Coventry suggested to local evaluators (Daly and Roebuck, 2008, p 21):

"The individual budget pilot has allowed [my] needs and aspirations to be understood in a way that a traditional assessment would not allow. In the past [my] ability to perform tasks would be the main focus of an assessment and the consequences of doing the task would not be considered."

In many ways, a similar message was to emerge from the national IBSEN evaluation (Glendinning et al, 2008, p 67), with 47% of people who accepted the offer of an individual budget suggesting that this had changed their view of what could be achieved in their lives 'a lot' (19% said 'a little'). For many of the early advocates of personal budgets, this was partly about enabling people to meet their needs more fully – but to do so in a way that makes sense for them and in a way that has the potential to connect people more fully to their friends, families and local communities.

Box 7.1: Achieving desired outcomes

Julia, a disabled parent, has used her individual budget to enable her to run a disabled people's organisation, to install air conditioning (which has prevented two hospital admissions) and to organise regular support to pick her son up from school.

Cyril and Beryl, both in their 80s, have used an individual budget to remain living in their own home. Instead of going into a care home for 'respite', they have been able to go to a hotel in Bournemouth and arrange support there (which was also cheaper than respite care).

Kate has a learning difficulty, and has used an individual budget to enable her to live independently and to access an IT course.

Frank is 91 and has used an individual budget to remain living in his own home. Although his family arranged support from a live-in care agency, the organisation concerned did not have a contract with the local social services and so could not have provided this support through the local authority. The individual budget enabled this existing arrangement to continue and prosper.

Cindy is registered blind and uses an individual budget to enable her to look after her young children (including going to mother and toddlers, doing the school run, shopping, housework and attending appointments etc).

Florence employs her granddaughter (a trained care worker). While her previous carers encouraged her to stop walking (for fear of a fall), her granddaughter has enabled her to walk again. In the DVD, the family are going to Longleat for the day.

Evangelos is the former manager of a travel agency and plans to use his individual budget to enable him to meet his personal care needs, but in a way that enables him to get out of his flat and socialise.

Elsie is 83 and uses an individual budget to get a regular bath at a local Age Concern centre (since her bathroom is inaccessible).

George has mental health problems and has used his individual budget to stay well and out of hospital. Instead of 'respite care', he went on holiday with a friend to Tunisia. He has also bought some painting materials in order to develop his interest in art (which is very different to the art he might do at a traditional mental health day centre).

Bob uses his individual budget to pay for practical support that helps him meet his personal care needs, but which also helps him work for a local disabled people's organisation. It has always been his ambition to go up in a hot-air balloon – while he has not yet managed this, the DVD shows him flying an aeroplane for the first time.

Angela is 92 and pays for her own live-in support. Her individual budget is used to pay for additional assistance in the evenings. Her overall support enables her to continue her life-long commitment to teaching and lecturing.

All personal stories taken from the *Living Your Life, Your Way* DVD (DH/Care Services Improvement Partnership/In Control, 2008).

Use of resources

Throughout the implementation of direct payments and personal budgets, issues of cost and of cost-efficiency have been paramount. While the possibility of direct payments legislation was being debated in Parliament, initial government opposition was based at least in part on fears about the cost implications of making payments to individuals instead of providing services (see Chapter Three). When direct payments were formally introduced, therefore, the accompanying guidance emphasised that:

> A local authority should not make direct payments unless they are at least as cost-effective as the services which it would otherwise arrange … (DH, 1997, p 16)

As a result, much of the research to date has included a consideration of value for money. In many cases, this has even happened in studies where the researchers do not appear to value cost-efficiency themselves, but feel the need to include a discussion of this issue because of its centrality to the government's agenda. For this reason, there is a substantial body of literature that suggests that direct payments are more cost-effective than directly provided services and, in some studies, may sometimes even be cheaper.

Certainly, this has been the case with the ILF, which has been found to be around 30% cheaper than direct services (quoted in Mandelstam, 1999, p 233). Prior to the implementation of direct payments, Morris wrote that 'enabling people to employ their own personal assistants is a more cost-effective way of meeting personal assistance needs than using local authority home care services' (Morris, 1993a, p 168). This assertion appeared to be based primarily on research conducted as part of an evaluation of the Personal Assistance Advisor post at Greenwich Association of Disabled People (Oliver and Zarb, 1992). Even when the cost of the support provided by the advisor was taken into account, the scheme still appeared to be cheaper than providing services directly. As Conservative minister,

Nicholas Scott, wrote in his foreword to the evaluation: 'This report on Personal Assistance Schemes in Greenwich shows that as well as being cost effective, such schemes offer disabled people a greater degree of independence when compared with traditional forms of provision' (Oliver and Zarb, 1992, Foreword).

Perhaps the most influential study was carried out by Zarb and Nadash (1994), specifically seeking to address issues of cost-efficiency in response to the then Conservative government's reluctance to legalise direct payments (see also Evans and Hasler, 1996). In order to compare the care packages of service users receiving some form of payment with those of people receiving direct services, the study sought to calculate unit costs for both types of support, taking account of all the expenditure involved. Although the methodology for compiling and comparing this data was complex, the researchers concluded that care packages financed by direct/indirect payments were, on average, some 30–40% cheaper than directly provided services (see Table 7.1). In addition to this, the researchers also noted that the concept of 'cost-efficiency' should incorporate not only issues of cost, but also a consideration of quality. That direct payments resulted in higher-quality services had already been demonstrated earlier in the study, where payment recipients suggested that:

- payment schemes met a wider range of needs than traditional services and led to fewer unmet needs;
- people receiving payments had more reliable support and experienced fewer problems with their care;
- payment recipients expressed higher levels of satisfaction than people using directly provided services.

Overall, the researchers were adamant that:

> Every pound spent through a payments scheme not only goes further than a pound spent on services, but also purchases assistance of a higher quality … Direct/indirect payments clearly represent better value for money than direct service provision. (Zarb and Nadash, 1994, p 143; see also Table 7.1 and Box 7.2).

Table 7.1: Average hourly unit costs

Type of care package	Average hourly unit costs of care
Direct/indirect payments	£5.18
Directly provided services	£8.52

Source: Zarb and Nadash, 1994, pp 117-43.

Box 7.2: Costs and benefits of direct payments

What the research evidence tells us is that direct payments have consistently been shown to be a cost-effective mechanism for enabling disabled people to access high-quality support that maximises choice and control at equivalent or, often, lower cost than other forms of community-based support. The most detailed study carried out in the UK, for example, showed that support packages based on direct payments were on average 30–40% cheaper than equivalent directly provided services. This study also highlighted very clearly that people receiving direct or indirect payments had higher overall levels of satisfaction with their support arrangements than service users. This was particularly noticeable in relation to reliability and flexibility and the degree of confidence that people had in their support arrangements being able to meet their needs.

Other smaller-scale studies have shown similar results. The evidence from this research demonstrates that user-controlled money goes further, so investing in independent living is a more cost-effective use of public finance.

(Zarb, 1998, p 1)

After the implementation of direct payments, research has continued to emphasise the cost–efficiency of paying money directly to disabled people. In West Sussex, a new direct payments scheme was reported to have made direct savings of £30,000 per year for just 15 recipients, while at the same time enabling them to purchase additional hours of care that would have cost £23,000 if delivered by in-house services (quoted in Hasler, 1999, p 7). In Scotland, research suggests that direct payments can lead to a more efficient use of human and financial resources, while also improving the quality and appropriateness of care (Witcher et al, 2000, para 7.8). In particular, the researchers found that time invested in setting up direct payments schemes can be recouped in the medium/long term, that direct payments can be cheaper than using agency care and that direct payments improve quality by enabling needs to be met more effectively. In Norfolk, it proved difficult to calculate some of the hidden costs associated with a direct payments scheme, but an evaluation still concluded that direct payments were a more cost-effective option than traditional services. This was despite the fact that the support arrangements in this particular scheme were extremely complex and that responsibility was split between two different agencies, thus duplicating a number of costs:

> Direct payments are a cheaper alternative than direct service provision or contracted agency services and become cheaper still comparatively over time ... It is difficult to envisage an alternative means of delivering a community care service ... which would be cheaper than a direct payments scheme. (Dawson, 2000, p 46)

Elsewhere, anecdotal evidence suggests that direct payments may *not* necessarily be cheaper than directly provided services, but *do* represent value for money. This is the opinion expressed by Roy Taylor, then director of community services for the Royal Borough of Kingston-upon-Thames and chair of the former ADSS Disabilities Committee. In a Department of Health (1998a) promotional video, Taylor warns against the assumption that direct payments will necessarily result in huge savings for local authorities, but does emphasise that:

- disabled people have shown themselves to be very innovative in designing care;
- disabled people are in control of their payments and want to use this money as effectively as possible;
- disabled people can often make better use of their payments than the local authority.

More recently, the growing literature continues to suggest that direct payments enable a more effective use of scarce resources – with opinion divided as to whether or not this actually reduces overall costs. In evidence submitted to the Wanless Review on the funding of older people's services, for example, Poole's (2006) analysis of direct payments and older people cites local evidence of potential savings, with one case study local authority reducing costs by around 17% of direct service costs (p 11). Elsewhere, the Audit Commission (2006) has suggested that introducing choice can lead to higher-quality services, increased control and greater user satisfaction, but that there is a trade-off to be made between start-up costs and any longer-term efficiency gains. While direct payments can cost more to set up and administer, the benefits can include greater flexibility, more empowered users and more appropriate care for minority groups. Having explored a series of different scenarios, the Audit Commission concludes that direct payments are likely to add to the cost of providing social care where direct payment rates are no lower than the cost of in-house provision. However, where direct payment rates *are* lower than in-house unit costs, there is scope for savings (which range in size depending on how many direct payment recipients there are and how much lower direct payments are than in-house unit costs). While this is probably not surprising, it means that there is a crucial trade-off to be made between the rate of direct payments, any savings that might occur and the extent to which the rate enables people to meet their needs (see Chapter Eight for further discussion).

Since the advent of personal budgets, the emerging evidence suggests that this way of working may also be more cost-effective than the previous system largely because it helps to unleash the creativity of people who have previously been passive recipients of services. In early In Control pilots, five case study authorities saved a minimum of 12% (see Poll et al, 2006). Elsewhere, Demos research in ten local authorities suggests a possible saving of around 10% (compared to the cost of traditional services). When excluding those people moved onto a personal budget because their needs and funding had both increased, the cost savings were closer to 15% (Leadbeater et al, 2008, pp 37–8). In the second phase of In Control (2005–07), detailed costings for 104 people who had previously used traditional social care prior to receiving a personal budget revealed a reduction in average costs by 9% (from £29,319 to £26,615) (Hatton et al, 2008, p 47). When people without prior experience of traditional social care were included, the figures fell further (by 15%, from £29,319 to £24,857). More recently, independent national evaluations confirm that personal budgets (and personal health budgets) are cost-effective (Glendinning et al, 2008; Forder et al, 2012 – although see Slasberg et al, 2012a–b, 2014 for an alternative view). Glendinning et al (2008, p 111), for example, conclude:

> Given the short follow-up for people allocated to the IB group and the delays in actual implementation – at the time of interview, some people did not have their support plans in place and for many others they had only been set up relatively recently – the findings are broadly encouraging for the new arrangements:

- Across *all user groups combined* there is some evidence that IBs are more cost-effective in achieving overall social care outcomes, but no advantage in relation to psychological well-being.
- For *people with learning disabilities*, there is a cost-effectiveness advantage in terms of social care outcomes but only really when we exclude people without support plans in place from the analysis. In other words, the *potential* is there to achieve cost-effectiveness, but implementation delays in the pilot sites meant that we did not observe this during the evaluation period. When looking at the psychological well-being outcome, standard care arrangements look slightly more cost-effective than IBs.
- Cost-effectiveness evidence in support of IBs is strongest for *mental health service users*, on both the outcome measures examined here.
- For *older people*, there is no sign of a cost-effectiveness advantage for either IBs or standard support arrangements using the social care outcomes measure. Using the General Health Questionnaire outcome measure, standard arrangements look marginally more cost-effective.
- There appears to be a small cost-effectiveness advantage for IB over standard support arrangements for younger physically disabled people using either of the outcome measures.

Similarly, Forder et al (2012, p 156) found that:

> The study suggested that personal health budgets are cost-effective, producing valued well-being benefits with a largely neutral impact on (recurrent) costs and on health/clinical outcomes.

While self-directed support might achieve savings in situations where people have high-cost packages of support, however, the former Audit Commission (2010) warned councils not to expect significant savings (see also Woolham and Benton, 2012 for additional discussion of costs and benefits in a case study local authority, and research by Wilberforce et al, 2011, 2012 into the impact on commissioning, market development and service providers). As with direct payments, therefore, this may be more about trying to use existing resources differently than it is about making active savings – and additional challenges will undoubtedly emerge as councils seek to roll out personal budgets more widely.

While these issues are complex and contested, a helpful conceptual contribution comes from an early In Control paper on 'The economics of self-directed support' (Duffy and Waters, 2008). Although this stresses that current data is incomplete, Duffy and Waters argue that the previous system is inherently inefficient because of the extent to which it is shaped by the pre-purchased services it has inherited from the past. This, it is claimed, leads to a potentially massive waste of resources, in a number of different ways (Duffy and Waters, 2008, pp 49–54).

- Resources are misdirected (as people have to have what there is rather than what they want or need).
- Multiple funding sources and assessment processes duplicate effort.
- The system forces people to inflate their needs in order to get help, and to play down their strengths and family networks.
- The current system rarely innovates, as decisions are taken too far away from the individuals they affect.
- There are very high transaction costs (perhaps as much as 30% of the current budget is spent in this way, including high spending on contracts and commissioning, care management and service management/administration and so on). However, it remains too early to know how much of this infrastructure is necessary and how much resource could be freed up in an era of self-directed support.

Quite what this means in practice is currently impossible to know, but remains (quite literally) the billion-dollar question. For some, self-directed support offers the opportunity to free up significant wasted resource in order to reinvest in meeting the needs of an ageing population, providing support to people with lower-level needs and investing in prevention. For others, this money could be reinvested in other priorities (essentially reducing the overall social care budget as money is moved elsewhere). For a third group, however, there is a potential counter-trend. As Duffy and Waters (2008, p 54) have argued:

> At present, the unattractiveness of the current social care system acts as a vicious form of rationing – rationing by not offering appropriate services. For some people, this lack of confidence in the quality of services acts as a significant deterrent ... If they can afford to stay away

from services … they do. However, when Self-Directed Support is available and authorities offer people choice, flexibility and control, 'new' eligible people [may] come forward and claim their right to a service.

This is also highlighted by Wilberforce et al (2012) in research into the impact of personal budgets on local authority commissioning and market development (p 255):

A final, unanswered question is whether commissioning budgets are at risk from demands from people eligible for services, but who had not previously taken these up. It has been argued that the prospect of a cash entitlement may encourage more people to do so … As such, personal budgets may become the victim of their own success; however whether this poses a genuine risk in England is not yet clear.

In many ways, this links back to the origins of social care (explored in Chapter Two), with 21st-century social care still operating a version of the principle of 'less eligibility' and 'the workhouse test'. While this raises questions that are beyond the scope of this book, the key issue is that the transparency of self-directed support holds out the potential for us to decide how much money to spend on adult social care as a society and how this is divided between people with support needs – irrespective of how much need and how much money there is out there, self-directed support allows us to take clear decisions about how best to respond to these challenges. Of course, a major irony here is that some supporters of self-directed support are so enthusiastic because of the financial transparency it brings, while some critics are hostile for exactly the same reason. Ultimately, perhaps, your view on whether or not transparency is a good thing probably depends on whether you think some of the rationing decisions we currently take should be open or hidden – and self-directed support goes right to the heart of this debate.

SUMMARY

Overall, direct payments and personal budgets seem to be two of the most powerful mechanisms available to transform the social care system, giving greater choice and control and delivering different and better outcomes for the same (or maybe even for less) money. As additional evidence has emerged, there has typically been a more cautious reaction to what is possible in practice – and both advocates and critics alike have been nervous about whether early potential positives can actually be sustained in such a difficult policy context. However, the fact remains that there is still much to celebrate and much to fight for – particularly if the underlying value base and ethos of direct payments and personal budgets can be maintained as they are mainstreamed and rolled out more systematically. For some people, direct payments and personal budgets 'just seem to work' – and the challenge for practitioners and policy makers may be how best to build on the potential positives and minimise the possible limitations now that both ways of working are national policy.

IMPLICATIONS FOR POLICY AND PRACTICE

- Direct payments and personal budgets offer greater choice and control to disabled people over their services and lives.
- This has the potential to improve morale and well-being – which could have a positive knock-on effect in a number of different ways.
- Being in control also enables people to make practical changes in their lives and to achieve outcomes that matter to them.
- Although opinion is divided, both direct payments and personal budgets seem to represent a more effective use of resources, since (at worst) they enable better outcomes to be achieved for the same amount of money.
- Outstanding issues include the extent to which a new system will encourage people with previously unidentified needs to come forward and/or the extent to which any direct savings can be reinvested in the system. Whether or not the former is a good thing or a bad thing might depend on your position within the system.

RECOMMENDED READING AND USEFUL WEBSITES

This chapter draws out key findings from more general material summarised in Chapters Three to Six, and so there are fewer further resources than in other chapters. As with Chapters Four and Five, some of the key overviews include:

- early national direct payment studies such as those by Riddell et al (2006), Vick et al (2006) and Davey et al (2007a–b);
- In Control evaluations (Poll et al, 2006; Hatton et al, 2008; Waters and Hatton, 2014);
- the national IBSEN evaluation (Glendinning et al, 2008; 2009) and the national evaluation of personal health budgets (Forder et al, 2012).

For discussion of the cost-effectiveness of direct payments, see Zarb and Nadash's (1994) pioneering early study. A helpful summary of the issues surrounding costs is available via In Control's paper on 'The economics of self-directed support' (Duffy and Waters, 2008), while the former Audit Commission (2010) provides a helpful analysis of the financial management of personal budgets (including consideration of value for money, resource allocation and subsequent commissioning strategies). Pearson et al (2014) seek to place the development of self-directed support in a broader public policy context by considering personalisation in an era of austerity (in particular ch 5).

REFLECTIVE EXERCISES
1. Keep a brief diary of the practical things you do during a single day – for example, getting up, getting washed, eating, going out of the house, working. How would your life change if you were reliant on directly provided services?
2. Continuing to reflect on this scenario, write a list of the pros and cons of directly provided services – and of direct payments/personal budgets. How might these different approaches act either as a facilitator or a barrier to living your life your way?
3. Talk to someone with experience of using services – and ask them the same questions. What is important to them about life and how does the support they receive help or hinder these aspirations?
4. Think about a time where you haven't been able to control or influence a situation (where you have been completely dependent on someone else). This could be an example from any walk of life. How did it make you feel? If the situation lasted for more than a short period, how did it affect you over time?
5. For people currently working in social care settings, how well do we spend existing resources? Are there ways in which direct payments/personal budgets might enable some of this scarce resource to be spent differently – or perhaps even better?

EIGHT

Possible barriers

This chapter explores:
- the different motives of those supporting direct payments and personal budgets;
- the barriers that can be created by some frontline workers;
- the consequences of inadequate funding levels;
- the danger of exacerbating inequity;
- gender and the impact on the workforce;
- issues of risk
- practical barriers (including staff recruitment).

As Chapter Seven demonstrated, direct payments and personal budgets bring a range of benefits that can enhance the choice, control and well-being of recipients. However, we have also seen how pressure for direct payments built up over a long period (Chapters Two and Three) and how organisations of disabled people were able to mount a sustained campaign for the new legislation to be introduced. As a result, direct payments were initially viewed positively by many people (and there were well-developed arguments built on years of experience and campaigning to answer the doubts of sceptics). Similarly, the speed and passion with which personal budgets have been developed and rolled out have sometimes meant that they have been promoted with significant enthusiasm – almost evangelically at times. While the arguments put forward have convinced a number of people (us included), this atmosphere has sometimes made it difficult to feel able to ask more difficult questions – and practitioners in particular tell us that they have a number of doubts that they do not feel able to share. We do not feel that this is a healthy situation – if people have concerns, then it is important that they feel able to be open about them and explore them with others.

While we believe that direct payments and personal budgets *do* bring a number of very real advantages, there have been a number of limitations and contradictions in practice that workers and service users need to consider. As Fernandez et al (2007) observe, many of these fall into one of two different categories:

- practical implementation barriers (which are capable, at least in principle, of being resolved by technical or management interventions);
- political, economic and social factors (which presumably require national and more fundamental change to resolve altogether).

While different accounts have tended to focus more on one or the other of these, the reality is that key barriers are likely to derive from a more complex mix of both factors. Against this background, this chapter seeks to explore a number of key questions, including:

- Are direct payments and personal budgets the product of a government seeking to restrict public spending and introduce a flawed notion of consumerism into community care services?
- Does the success of direct payments and personal budgets rely too heavily on the attitudes and training of front-line workers?
- Are direct payments and personal budgets adequately financed, and do recipients receive enough money to purchase sufficient care?
- Could direct payments and personal budgets introduce a two-tier system, leaving people who receive direct services in a disadvantageous position and/or enabling those with the loudest voice/the greatest family support to get better outcomes?
- Might direct payments and personal budgets lead to the greater exploitation of care workers and of women?
- Could direct payments and personal budgets leave service users vulnerable to abuse or at risk of significant harm?
- Are the practicalities of managing direct payments and personal budgets prohibitive?

Consumerism and public expenditure

Although direct payments offer increased choice and control, it is often forgotten that they were introduced by a Conservative government firmly committed to New Right or neoliberal social and economic policies. Building on the work of thinkers such as Hayek (1944), Friedman (1962) and Murray (1984), the New Right approach has been summarised in terms of a belief in three key issues:

- the free market
- the minimal state
- individual liberty and responsibility. (Adams, 1998, p 85)

Within social policy, this has led to a neoliberal critique of state welfare that acquired increasing significance after the economic crises and political polarisation of the 1970s. As Alcock (1996, p 12) explains:

> [The New Right's] main argument was that state intervention to provide welfare services ... merely drove up the cost of public expenditure to a point where it began to interfere with the effective operation of a market economy. They claimed that this was a point that had already been reached in Britain in the 1970s as the high levels of taxation needed for welfare services had reduced profits, crippled investment and driven capital overseas. [At the same time]

the New Right also challenged the desirability of state welfare in practice, arguing that free welfare services only encouraged feckless people to become dependent upon them and provided no incentive for individuals and families to protect themselves through savings or insurance. Furthermore, right-wing theorists claimed that state monopoly over welfare services reduced the choices available to people to meet their needs in a variety of ways and merely perpetuated professionalism and bureaucracy.

After the election of Margaret Thatcher as prime minister in 1979, these ideas acquired increasing support at the heart of central government, culminating in a series of market-led reforms in traditional public sector services such as education, housing and the NHS. Within community care, such reforms were to transform social services departments from direct service providers into service purchasers, with an explicit brief to contract a significant amount of care from the independent sector (Lewis, 1996). These changes were presented as 'promoting choice and independence' and giving 'people a greater individual say in how they live their lives and the services they need to help them do so' (DH, 1989, p 4). This has been described by Means and Smith (1998a, p 83) as promoting a form of 'empowerment by exit':

> 'Exit' is essentially a market approach which seeks to empower consumers by giving them a choice between alternatives and the option of 'exit' from a service and/or provider, if dissatisfied. The consumer, in other words, will be able to change provider, and if a large number of them make the same decision about the same provider then that provider will be punished for their inefficiency by going out of 'business'.

Although neoliberal attempts to recast service users as consumers have led to greater emphasis on service quality, a consumerist approach to social policy has been criticised by a number of commentators (see, for example, Barnes and Walker, 1996; Means and Smith, 1998a). As Marian Barnes (1997, p 3) has suggested, empowerment by exit and the consumerist philosophy on which this is based both rely on a number of essential preconditions:

- Alternatives need to exist.
- The person concerned needs access to information not only about alternatives, but also about characteristics of alternatives that might suggest that they would overcome dissatisfaction with existing services, but also not substitute new for existing problems.
- Moving from one option to another should be practically possible.
- Moving from one option to another should not of itself generate damaging disruption.

As Barnes continues: 'If one considers the circumstances in which most people use health and social care services, it is clear that all these circumstances will rarely apply.'

In addition to promoting the notion of welfare recipients as consumers, the New Right also emphasised the need to curtail public spending on welfare. As we have seen in Chapter Two, the ILF introduced in 1988 was restricted in 1993 as a result of concerns about rapidly increasing costs. We have also seen in Chapters Two and Three how financial concerns thwarted previous attempts to introduce direct payments in the early 1990s and how government guidance emphasised the need for direct payments to be at least as cost-effective as the services that they replaced. Although the Community Care (Direct Payments) Act 1996 was introduced three years after the reform of the ILF, this was seen as less of a financial threat to the government, since direct payments were to be operated by local authorities within their existing cash-limited budgets (Means and Smith, 1998a, p 85). As the number of direct payments increased over time, moreover, there was evidence of a 'north–south divide' (Pearson, 2004, p 4), with Conservative strongholds in southern England more likely to adopt direct payments than areas associated more with 'Old' Labour politics.

More recently, similar concern about financial risk seems to have accompanied debates about personal budgets, and at least some of the current policy enthusiasm seems to come from the perception that this may be a way of responding to the needs of a rapidly ageing population without investing what many would see as the necessary resources (see Chapters Five to Seven for further discussion). Thus, as Henwood and Hudson (2007b) have demonstrated, some of the enthusiasm for personal budgets may have come from a range of different perspectives, with some keen to cut costs, some eager to transform the public perception of social care and others concerned about the role of social welfare in promoting or undermining independence. Described as 'a Holy Trinity of support', this prompted one respondent in the study to comment that, if so many apparently different people find the concept attractive, "then we may all be thinking it is something rather different" (Henwood and Hudson, 2007b, p 34).

Against this background, the introduction of direct payments and of personal budgets begins to take on a new and slightly more sinister appearance. While direct payments undoubtedly bring a number of very real benefits, it is also possible to see them as an attempt to promote a flawed notion of 'empowerment by exit' and to do so in a way that would not result in an escalation of public expenditure. In such a scenario, it would be left to local authorities to balance the books and reconcile the very real demand for direct payments with already stringent budget constraints. While this should not prevent service users from benefiting from the many advantages of direct payments and personal budgets, it does suggest that there may be conflicting agendas, with service users and central government each wanting different things from the reforms. This contradiction has been identified most forcefully by Pearson (2000, 2004), who has emphasised the tensions between the social justice discourse of the disability movement and the market discourse of government. In the same way, Askheim (2003) argues that those apparently committed to the notion of 'empowerment' can support the concept either from a market-based consumer stance, or from a radical civil rights perspective. This is further developed by Spandler (2004, p 190), who describes direct payments as 'a complex confluence of new right, New Labour and welfare user movement ideologies and demands', with scope to mask a range of underlying tensions and conflicts. As Fernandez et al (2007, p 99) argue:

> The policy appeals across the political spectrum ... Conservative commentators can applaud its market-like characteristics, while for New Labour the policy resonates neatly with the broader thrust of the choice in public services campaign ... The policy also seems to be remarkably popular with those users who have secured access to it.

Whether this is a good or a bad thing probably depends on your point of view. However, as Spandler (2004) observes, what would be dangerous is to assume common interests and to deny the existence of conflict – this will only reduce the impact of direct payments and personal budgets, prompting polarised responses and undermining critical discussion of the underlying issues. For front-line workers, moreover, such tensions may ultimately lead to role conflict as they try to support direct payment and personal budget recipients, while working within a system and within financial constraints that are not always as emancipatory as the initial policy rhetoric may suggest. Elsewhere, we have developed these arguments further (Glasby, 2012b), suggesting that the initial campaigns for change that surrounded direct payments and personal budgets involved some potentially very uneasy bedfellows coming together, often with very different motivations and expectations. While this created enough momentum to change policy, it remains to be seen what happens next if different groups with different values really do begin to diverge significantly. As Spandler (2004, p 202) suggests:

> Having explored some of the complexities ... it seems clear that neither a simplistic pursuit of [direct payments] as empowerment, nor a kneejerk reaction against them as mere cost-cutting consumerism is an adequate response. [Direct payments] are not clearly a 'consumerist' or a 'democratic' approach to social policy ..., but actually an example of the convergence of the two, a convergence that yields both problems and possibilities.

Similarly, as Sapey and Pearson (2004, p 65) suggest:

> Direct payments do make use of free market principles and there can be a contradiction between the individualism of this approach and the need for collectivity in the responsibility for welfare ... Direct payments need to be seen as an integral part of a collective approach

to the provision of support. Implementing direct payment schemes provides a possibility of promoting independent living and access to mainstream economic and social life, but also could become a threat to collective responsibility for welfare and the notion of caring communities if it is interpreted within an individualist framework. The challenge is to do the first and not the second.

More recently, these arguments have gained even greater significance in an age of austerity and under the Coalition government of 2010–15. As Duffy (2014) argues, the severe cuts which have been faced by disabled people constitute an 'unexpected reverse' (p 179) and raise even more fundamental questions about what might be needed next:

> The goal of personalisation was the advancement of citizenship. However, the means by which this goal was achieved was by the redesign of professional systems of control. In a sense, personalisation tried to change the Professional Gift Model into a Citizenship Model by stealth – by changing processes to encourage people to treat each other more like fellow citizens.

> But today … I wonder whether citizenship can ever really be achieved by stealth – simply by redesigning systems and processes. Indeed, historically, the battles for citizenship (from ancient Athens to women's suffrage, from a free India to black civil rights) have always been waged by citizens themselves – in their own name.

A similar point is raised by Beresford (2011/12, p 40), who contrasts the empowering nature of direct payments with what he feels has happened in practice more recently:

> From a means to empowerment [i.e. direct payments], we have moved to what is essentially an under-funded voucher system. From a replacement for a traditional and inadequate set of services, we have moved to an exchange relationship, which casts the service user as a consumer, not a citizen with rights – to a model that is market based and market driven rather than liberatory in intent. Of course personal budgets may still benefit some service users. This would not be difficult, unfortunately, given the poor quality of much traditional social care provision. But that is not what we were promised. We were promised something much better for *all* and that is not happening.

The 'gatekeeping' role of social workers

Time and time again, a major barrier to an extension of direct payments has been shown to be the attitudes and knowledge of front-line social workers. This was widely anticipated as the 1996 Act was being implemented (Oliver and Sapey, 1999), and subsequent events have tended to support those uncertain about the capacity of social services departments to embrace the significant changes implied by direct payments legislation. In Scotland, practitioners were deterred by perceived expenditure and workload implications, by a lack of understanding of direct payments, or by a fear of a loss of control (Witcher et al, 2000). Others feared that service users would misspend their payments on drugs or alcohol, and there was a widespread suggestion that senior managers may be deliberately 'blocking' the implementation of the 1996 legislation. Overall, understanding of direct payments was limited, with some departments unsure of the differences between direct and indirect payments.

Elsewhere (Fruin, 2000, p 17), the former Social Services Inspectorate found evidence of an ambivalent attitude to direct payments among staff:

> "I am very worried about direct payments – vulnerable people managing their own services." (Social worker in a multi-disciplinary team)

> "Can I risk [direct payments] ... on behalf of clients?" (Adults' team social worker)

Some members of staff lacked knowledge about direct payments legislation and about local procedures, disadvantaging their service users. In the local inspections, direct payments sometimes had a low profile among non-specialist workers and might not be adequately publicised, through fears that this would create additional demands on already stretched budgets. On one occasion, proposals for a direct payments scheme were hindered by the lack of a champion to drive forward the project and a lack of understanding about the role that direct payments could play in the range of services designed to support independent living (DH/SSI, 1999a–c). Similar findings were also to emerge from Norfolk (Dawson, 2000) and Staffordshire, where an evaluation of a direct payments pilot project emphasised the need to promote awareness not only among disabled people, but also among social workers (Leece, 2000, pp 39–40). In West Sussex, social workers were found to have very little knowledge of direct payments, with some practitioners claiming that people with learning difficulties could not receive direct payments but that disabled children could (quoted in Leece, 2000, p 39). Findings such as these supported previous research in London that suggested that people at all levels – users, carers and junior members of staff – had little knowledge of direct payments (Brandon et al, 2000; Maglajlic et al, 2000). In the case of people with learning difficulties, interviews with ten users, ten carers and ten members of staff found that only two members of staff out of the 30 people interviewed had even heard of direct payments (Maglajlic et al, 2000, pp 100–1). For older people, research carried out by Age Concern suggested that few staff within social services knew anything about direct payments (even in areas with a history of them), raising serious questions as to how service users were to be kept informed (Age Concern, 1998; see also Box 8.1).

Box 8.1: Lack of information

"The information that gets here is lousy. Sometimes they tell you something, like 'you can have this' ... And then they say that it's going to be in two months, three months ... and then you hear nothing else about it."

(Quoted in Maglajlic et al, 2000, p 101)

"My social worker had difficulty accessing relevant information. Her manager did not have the answers to her questions and could not tell her where to find the answer."

(Quoted in Leece, 2000, p 39)

Despite widespread information campaigns, many people with learning difficulties still know nothing about direct payments.

(Bewley, 2000, p 14)

As the Direct Payments pilot project progressed, it became increasingly apparent that the single most significant factor in determining who became an employer through direct payments was the potential employer's social worker.

(Dawson, 2000, p 22)

Elsewhere, it may not just be lack of knowledge that hinders implementation, but political and/or professional opposition. Depending on the political views of local councillors and social services managers, some authorities may view direct payments as a threat to their own in-house domiciliary and day care (George, 1996), representing a form of 'privatisation by the back door' (Hasler et al, 1999, p 7). At the same time, direct payments might be expected to lead to a change in social work practice, prompting a shift away from providing/purchasing services for disabled people, and toward supporting them to purchase their own care. This feature of direct payments is particularly identified by Dawson (2000) in her evaluation of the Norfolk Independent Living Project. During the study, it became apparent that a significant majority of people without previous experience of indirect payment schemes had heard of direct payments through their social worker, but that some practitioners were withholding this information. Whereas staff specialising in work with people with physical impairments were familiar with the concept of indirect payments, workers from mental health or learning difficulty teams had little knowledge of users purchasing their own care. As the evaluation progressed, it became clear that the introduction of direct payments involved 'a change of culture' in which individual workers were having to take on more of an enabling role (Dawson, 2000, p 53). While some staff relished this role, others were less enthusiastic, and the take-up of direct payments was directly linked to the approach of individual workers (see Box 8.2).

Box 8.2: The role of care management

My involvement in the promotion of direct payments does raise questions for me about the current state of play in care management. Care managers are extremely important gatekeepers in the whole direct payments story. I have a strong impression that people with learning difficulties who have been able to access direct payments have always had a champion on their side. This has often been a forward-thinking (and tenacious) family member, independent advisor, advocate or, sometimes, care manager. These care managers have been vital in the promotion of direct payments so far, but they are not the majority within social services. If direct payments are to become an easy mainstream option ... then enabling people to access them must become normal care management practice. For this to happen, significant change is required to individual, team and organisational practice around care management ... The care management system is under many pressures and the truth is that direct payments are not a daily priority for many care managers ... This is a shame because the ethos of direct payments is extremely exciting. Care managers now have the chance to actually give service users the money to buy their own services. This sharing of power, this chance to see individual lives flourish whilst practical support needs are met, is a fantastic opportunity for care managers to be inspired by their job. The opportunity is there.

(Bewley, 2000, pp 14–15)

In one sense, such barriers might have been expected (especially given the scale of the cultural challenge that direct payments imply). Unfortunately, this does not yet seem to be something that is going away; perceived resistance from front-line staff remains a key feature of the more recent direct payments literature. According to a survey of direct payment support services, for example, resistance from staff was the second most frequently cited barrier to direct payments (Davey et al, 2007a, p 83), while CSCI (2004) has placed similar emphasis on the potentially negative impact that a lack of meaningful information and support from care managers can have. At local level, Clark and Spafford (2002) have demonstrated how many workers found it hard to take ownership of this new way of working due to time/work pressures, anxieties about how to offer direct payments in a meaningful way, concerns about interpreting the guidance on being 'willing and able', tensions between promoting empowerment and balancing risk, and concerns about flexibility for some versus equity for all. As some of the participants in the study commented:

> "We don't need this; we've already got enough hassle, do we need any more hassle?"

> "It's daunting to offer something that you don't fully understand yourself."

> "You lose your autonomy ... it's like the symbol of wearing a badge to say you're a professional and then suddenly the badge disappears, 'Ah, they won't know what I am'."

(Clark and Spafford, 2002, pp 250, 252)

However, a particularly vivid description of the role of social workers in influencing people's access to direct payments comes from Ellis's (2007) study of assessment and care management practice in one English local authority. While Ellis argues that direct payments might be able to help social workers re-engage with the core values of the profession, the realities of front-line practice (especially time and financial constraints) meant that practitioners often rationed access to direct payments by a variety of informal means. These included introducing the concept in a defensive manner, restricting access to information, focusing on assessment and simply leaving a leaflet about direct payments, or making assumptions about the 'right sort of person' for a direct payment. Such tactics were justified in a range of ways (see Box 8.3), and Ellis's study provides a fascinating insight into the subconscious processes that can sometimes make us adopt particular critiques of a specific policy as a way of justifying how we respond to the pressures of the workplace. Interestingly, the language employed by many of the participants in this study also serves as confirmation of the continued dominance of Duffy's 'professional gift' model (see Chapters Two and Five), with workers often using words such as 'let', 'allow' and 'give' in relation to their role in working with service users (Ellis, 2007, p 418).

In many ways, the crucial role of social workers in encouraging or preventing disabled people to access direct payments is hardly surprising. Previous research into the information provided by social services departments has suggested that inefficient distribution systems and poor targeting can prevent information from reaching the right people at the right time and in the right place. Although many authorities produce material in different formats and languages, most information has historically been in standard print (Fryer, 1998). Even where authorities make considerable efforts to produce accessible information for minority groups, the publicity and leaflets that do exist may not always find their way to the people who need them (DH/SSI, 1997). For disabled people trying to make sense of the

Box 8.3: 'Justifications' for rationing access to direct payments

In legitimising their rationing of access to direct payments, social workers put forward a number of 'justifications' (Ellis, 2007), including:

- the perception that direct payments meet 'wants' rather than 'needs' – that they are optional extras above and beyond the core business of current social care;
- the belief that direct payments enable people to meet their needs in non-traditional ways, and this could be inequitable for recipients of directly provided services;
- concerns about financial abuse.

While these are all potentially legitimate concerns (albeit ones to which we think there are very robust answers), Ellis's study is especially helpful as it highlights the way in which the pressures of front-line practice can hinder the offering of direct payments, with the practitioners concerned citing such factors not necessarily because there are genuine barriers, but in order to justify the stance they feel forced to take by practice realities.

complexities of social services bureaucracy, the difficulty of obtaining accessible information about the options open to them has been well documented (see Box 8.4; Beardshaw, 1988; Zarb and Oliver, 1993; Barnes, 1995; Davis et al, 1997). In one research project, two case study social services departments were not providing disabled people with the information and advice they needed, since front-line staff saw requests for information as potential demands on their services (Davis et al, 1997). Elsewhere, the Social Services Inspectorate found that information for disabled people could be out of date and repetitive, not specific to disabled people, inaccessible to people from minority ethnic groups and poorly distributed (DH/SSI, 1996). Even after direct payments became mandatory rather than discretionary, there is still a key role for front-line staff in communicating the different options as positively as possible, so as not to bias service users and artificially constrain choice. As one participant in a national study of the implementation of direct payments observed:

> "What I am concerned about is *how* people are being offered it. If it's presented as a positive alternative, people are more likely to take it up, but if it is not sold to hard to reach client groups, they won't touch it ... Teams are becoming aware that it is mandatory, however it still comes down to the social worker and selling direct payments and there is a block here, they don't feel confident and are lacking info. Making it mandatory has helped a bit but it hasn't dealt with the problem." (Vick et al, 2006, p 33)

As the quote above begins to suggest, it has long been recognised that social workers occupy a crucial gatekeeping role and can work in a number of informal ways to limit the demands made upon them (Rees, 1978; Satyamurti, 1981).

Described by Lipsky (1980) as 'street level bureaucrats', social workers have been shown to use their professional discretion in order to balance competing priorities and to protect themselves against the overwhelming pressures that they face (see Box 8.5). Often, they will seek to manage their workloads by making assumptions about their service users, categorising them and forming stereotypical responses to their needs, thereby adding a degree of stability and predictability to their work. Although the concept of street-level bureaucracy was initially applied to the reorganisation of social services departments in the 1970s, research funded by the JRF has demonstrated that front-line practitioners continue to behave in similar ways (Davis et al, 1997; Ellis et al, 1999). Based on observations of social work assessments and interviews with users and carers, the study found that workers used screening mechanisms, computer-based assessments and eligibility criteria to manage demand, thereby rationing their time and resources. Although the methods of rationing would appear to have changed since the 1970s, the gatekeeping role of social workers is just as real. Against this background, the success of direct payments is likely to continue to be closely linked to the attitudes and actions of front-line staff, and it will be important to ensure that practitioners receive sufficient information and training to be able to become forces for change rather than obstacles to progress.

Box 8.4: Access to information

Information is also a key pre-requisite to disabled people having genuine choice and control over how their needs are to be met. Without information about available resources, how to access services, or about their rights, it is impossible for people to make genuine choices or determine what kind of support is most appropriate to meet their self-defined needs. However, previous research has often highlighted information poverty as a major constraint on providing appropriate and adequate solutions to disabled people's support needs.

(Zarb and Oliver, 1993, p 9)

Box 8.5: Street-level bureaucracy

The decisions of street-level bureaucrats, the routines they establish, and the devices they invent to cope with uncertainties and work pressures, effectively become the public policies they carry out ... Public policy is not best understood as made in legislatures or top-floor suites of high-ranking administrators, because in important ways it is actually made in the crowded offices and daily encounters of street-level workers.

(Lipsky, 1980, p xii)

With the advent of personal budgets, the issues at stake arguably become even more profound. While personal budgets start to overcome some of the practical concerns that front-line workers have raised about direct payments (for example, that some user groups would find administering their payments too onerous and that payments could not be used for public services), the move to a system of self-directed support requires a radical rethink of the nature of modern social work. Under self-directed support, the role of the local authority is to allocate a financial resource to the individual, then to check that the support plans they are making seem sensible and that the needs for which the personal budget is provided are being met. Thus, the focus shifts from the current very heavy emphasis on assessment, to support planning and review – almost reversing current practice. In addition, the role of social workers is to support those people without access to other forms of support or those who want a social worker to help manage their personal budget. While some see this as undermining the professional status of social workers, others see it very much as freeing up extremely skilled and experienced staff to concentrate on those people who need them most – essentially enabling social workers to do what they came into the job to do in the first place (see Glendinning et al, 2008, Chapter 12 for evidence of both views). Certainly, this was the line taken by New Labour, with a paper on the workforce implications of *Putting People First* stating that:

> Achieving [policy aspirations for adult social care] … relies on the capacity, competency and commitment of the social care workforce … to empower and support people who use services and supports to exercise that choice and control. It will mean a workforce assuming a more proactive and enabling role in how they respond to people's needs and preferences but having far less control over the details of the support that people receive – taking on roles which strongly focus on brokerage, information and service advocacy. It will mean less direct management control over people's lives by social care professionals, but still ensuring they carry out their duty to care. It will mean embracing new ways of working when it comes to identifying and responding to risk and becoming less risk averse. *This is not a relinquishing of responsibility: it is working in a true partnership between social care workers and people using services, their carers, those who volunteer and the wider community. Such partnership working is, we know, why so many people decided to become social care professionals in the first place.* (DH, 2008d, pp 4–5, emphasis added)

While this is a stance with which we fully agree, the evidence from direct payments suggests that substantial training and development may be required in order to persuade front-line staff that this is indeed the case. Without this, personal budgets could struggle with the same cultural challenges as direct payments, and their impact could be weakened. Early on, moreover, there is evidence to suggest that the introduction of new ways of working can increase rather than reduce workloads (Wilberforce et al, 2014), with staff having to operate the old and new systems at the same time (Glendinning et al, 2008, ch 12). While some of this may reduce over time as new ways of working become more established, it is interesting to note that Hasler and Marshall's (2013) summary of the barriers to increasing the take-up of direct payments – some 17 years after the initial Community Care (Direct Payments) Act 1996 – lists only five barriers for professionals (all of which are primarily attitudinal/cultural):

- 'Low staff awareness…
- Lack of training…
- Restrictive or patronising attitudes about the capabilities of people who might use a direct payment and a reluctance to devolve power away from professionals to people who use the service
- Reluctance to refer people to User Led Organisations
- Fears/assumptions that disabled people will not be able to manage (particularly older people and people with mental health problems' (p 4).

To date, the signs remain mixed. While there has been enthusiastic engagement with self-directed support in some areas, a number of barriers still remain (see Glendinning et al, 2008 for a summary; see also Mickel, 2008). Although this is very much an oversimplification, battlelines have often seemed to be drawn between personal budget recipients and their allies, on the one hand, and some social care professional bodies and broader public service trade unions, on the other (see Box 8.6 for examples). While some of the short-term tensions between these two groups have undoubtedly been increased by the scale and pace of reform, it seems a shame that all stakeholders involved in the delivery and receipt of social care do not currently seem able to find common ground and a shared value base. Although this is perhaps to be expected with such fundamental changes, social care workers and people who receive services both have very few allies, and it would be unfortunate if the whole of social care cannot work together to tackle some of these issues.

This is clearly complex and disputed territory, but a paper by In Control provides a helpful summary of many of the key issues (Duffy, 2007). In particular, Duffy identifies three limitations of previous approaches to care management:

- *The inflexibility of the resources that are available to identify and meet need*: although the early advocates of care management envisaged significant flexibility, many care managers find that they have to rely heavily on existing block-contracted services and thus have little discretion to meet needs in other ways.
- *The disguised nature of the rationing system by which resources are assigned*: while the care management guidance required social workers to operate within appropriate budgets, the process of rationing has tended to lack transparency (with the result that workers can feel a conflict of interest between supporting

Box 8.6: Tensions in the social care workforce

As an example of those passionate about the potentially liberating impact of direct payments and personal budgets, Simon Stevens (an independent disability trainer and consultant, and regular columnist in *Community Care* magazine) has argued that:

> My attempts to quell my feelings about trade unions have not been successful. After realising that a system in which personal assistants are paid by disabled micro-employers is likely to be the way forward, they appear to have decided to abandon rational debate. Instead, they are beginning to spread 'caveman-style' propaganda that disabled people are naturally bad employers who will disobey their legal duties and abuse their staff ... This is an interesting opening standpoint in what is clearly going to be a long and bloody battle between the rights of service users and indeed their staff with the demands of an external self-appointed 'god', making judgements on highly complex issues about which they have little understanding. I strongly believe that if my staff were forced to join a trade union, I would be better off dead.

(Stevens, 2008)

Shortly afterwards, a Scottish study by Unison was presented in the trade press as being critical of the workforce implications of self-directed support:

> Personalised support schemes are breaching the employment rights of care assistants, Unison has warned. A Scottish study by the union found that some employees were failing to benefit from the minimum wage, statutory leave or maternity pay. Evidence from self-directed support schemes in Scotland showed care assistants hired by disabled people using personal budgets worked under conditions which broke employment law.

(Lombard, 2008)

Leaving aside the detail of these two stances, the way in which both were reported (and the reaction they generated) is probably more important than the original column and research study – what this suggests is that finding common ground in a way that brings people needing support together with those who provide it can be difficult, and that the issues can quickly become polarised if we do not focus sufficiently on the underlying principles and goals of self-directed support.

the person and balancing the books, and that access to resources can often depend on the extent to which individual workers can advocate on behalf of 'their' client).

- *The professionally dominated process of planning and organising support*: at present, care managers are meant to assess, develop care plans and organise support for all – irrespective of the capacities, networks and gifts of the individuals concerned. Interestingly, when approximately 100 care managers were asked who was the best person to plan and organise support for people on their current caseloads (around 800 cases), they often chose other people (family, friends, service providers or the person themselves) rather than a care manager (see Duffy, 2007, p 7).

In contrast, Duffy argues, self-directed support makes the allocation of resources to meet need transparent, improves support planning and frees up care managers to focus their skills on those who need them most. As one personal budget project manager observed:

> "Generally speaking, the introduction of [personal budgets] has been met with considerable enthusiasm and commitment by practitioners ..., principally because of the focus on user empowerment and creativity in support planning. Many practitioners and team managers feel that this is 'what real social work is about ... it's what I trained for'." (Quoted in Duffy, 2007, p 11)

In addition to In Control material on this issue, one of the most insightful commentaries on the scale of the cultural challenge that accompanies self-directed support comes from Henwood and Hudson's (2007b) review of progress in three case study local authorities. As the researchers conclude, 'If [self-directed support] is to become established there has to be an understanding of its professional and organisational ramifications, otherwise – rather like the history of direct payments – it will tend to be seen as a marginal activity bolted on to existing arrangements' (Henwood and Hudson, 2007b, p 14; see also Box 8.7). In particular, Henwood and Hudson identify a series of cultural challenges that will need to be overcome for self-directed support to be successfully implemented, including:

- the culturally conservative nature of social care, with many social care organisations seen as 'not well-suited to radical change' (p 15);
- the difficulties in supporting current care managers to take on new roles and become fully committed to the new system;
- a history of 'giving and doing' (p 20), with a workforce that measures itself by its ability to do things *for* people and give them services;
- fears that self-directed support could lead to an overly individual approach and threaten collective social welfare;
- concerns that self-directed support could end up meeting 'wants' rather than 'needs';
- a tendency for some front-line workers to mistrust service users and carers (with implicit assumptions that significant input from professionals is required to safeguard public money);
- assumptions that older people would not want the perceived complexities associated by some participants with self-directed support.

> ## Box 8.7: The cultural challenges of self-directed support
>
> "We are often tempted to change processes rather than behaviours. This is about changing a set of behaviours – process and legislation is a second-order issue. For me this is about a change in mindset."
>
> "I am generalising, but I don't think the penny has dropped yet. People think they can do it as an add-on. Unless work is actively done quite soon we are going to struggle to implement this."
>
> "There is sometimes resistance from social workers who aren't sure they came into social work to provide money to people."
>
> "Most people totally agree with the principles but are wary that it will undermine their role. They are saying will there be a need for social workers and that 'we are professionally qualified for a reason'."
>
> (Staff reactions, Henwood and Hudson, 2007b, pp 14–18)

As Henwood and Hudson (2007b, p 26) observe:

> What much of the above ... reveals is a stark interpretation of [self-directed support] – an 'all or nothing' model in which the service user either takes the full package unaided or sticks with the current arrangements. It suggests that there needs to be a greater emphasis upon [self-directed support] as a continuum of options, as well as on the availability of personalisation support mechanisms.

Arising out of this analysis, Henwood and Hudson identify 'a variety of understandings and views' about self-directed support (2007b, p 27), dividing participants in their study into one of three different categories that may prove helpful when seeking to implement self-directed support locally:

- outright supporters – who fully understand and are committed to the principles of self-directed support;
- qualified supporters – who may support the overall principle but have some concerns;
- 'the confused and the critics' (p 29) – who either do not understand self-directed support or are hostile to it (or both).

Since this early contribution, there may well be a fourth group emerging – those who were initially supportive but who feel let down in practice by an innovation that has sometimes been implemented badly in a difficult policy context and therefore failed to deliver at local level. This is covered in greater detail in Chapter Six (see also Duffy, 2012a, 2012b, 2014), but 'the disillusioned' might well be a fourth category not initially identified in 2007 by Henwood and Hudson.

Financial difficulties

The financial implications of making cash payments to disabled people are an issue that has continued to be debated throughout the campaign for direct payments and beyond (see Chapter Seven for further discussion). We have also already seen how the motives of central government may have been influenced by a neoliberal belief in rolling back the welfare state and how concerns about public expenditure thwarted a series of early attempts to legalise direct payments in the early 1990s (Chapter Three). There is now a growing consensus that financial concerns may be a major obstacle to the success and progress of direct payments, preventing some local authorities from promoting their schemes and potentially leaving recipients with insufficient funds to purchase adequate care. This has since been exacerbated by a series of deep cuts in local government budgets and beyond, leaving people receiving welfare benefits, accessing social care and with housing needs facing something of a 'triple whammy' as the cuts bite.

In the early days, a key barrier to the implementation of direct payments may have been a lack of pump-priming to establish schemes with an appropriate support infrastructure (Wellard, 1999). Direct payments may be more cost-effective than direct services when a successful scheme is up and running, but there were workload and cost implications in seeking to set up such schemes in the first place. In many cases, early direct payment schemes were financed from generic community care budgets, with no additional funding. For departments already struggling to manage overstretched budgets, this was often a major disincentive to promoting direct payments as an option for disabled people. As one director of social services commented: "There won't be any extra provision in the revenue support grant, and direct payments could in fact attract more people into community care and so create additional demand. This could lead to delays in community care assessments, which are already a problem in many places" (quoted in George, 1996, p 24). Unfortunately, this was an issue that was identified as a potential problem from the very beginning:

> Funding could also prove to be a problem ... The pump priming and on-going revenue we have asked for shows little sign of materialising. This is an issue on which we will need to pitch hard during the expenditure round ... If the goal is to extend basic direct payments schemes on a widespread basis then pump priming will be necessary. If pressure for an even greater coverage becomes intense, then significant additional funds may be needed. (Taylor, 1996c, pp 9–10)

Elsewhere, there was evidence of considerable financial implications in an evaluation carried out in Norfolk (Dawson, 2000). Although direct payment packages were found to be cheaper than directly provided services, this comparison did not take account of a number of 'hidden costs' during the early stages of the direct payments scheme. In this particular case study, implementing direct payments required management time, a seconded worker to reassess people transferring from a previous third-party scheme and a range of consultative and team meetings (see Box 8.8). Negotiations were also extremely complex, requiring a commitment from senior management and considerable partnership working with a range of disability groups. Although the majority of these start-up costs were incurred early on in the scheme and might be expected to decrease as direct payments became more firmly established, the investment required to implement a direct payments scheme did have financial implications that may have concerned some local authorities.

Box 8.8: Hidden costs

Cost of direct payments, 1999–2000:	£735,867
Estimated cost of equivalent services:	£764,560
Hidden costs:	Management time
	A seconded worker
	Consultation
	Team meetings
	Negotiating and setting up support services
	Establishing system for monitoring and payment

(Adapted from Dawson, 2000, pp 43–4)

If financial concerns can create difficulties for local authorities, they can also be detrimental to direct payment recipients. Prior to the implementation of direct payments, Morris (1993a) revealed how indirect payment schemes and ILF contributions often failed to take account of indirect costs (including extra expenditure on food, entertainment and transport when being accompanied by a PA, as well as the costs of being an employer). For many people, this not only meant that such expenses had to come out of other income, but also contributed to bad employment practices, such as employing assistants on a cash-in-hand basis and failing to take out appropriate insurance. Hardly surprisingly, such issues were of particular concern to organisations such as the United Kingdom Home Care Association, which expressed its fears that the subsequent introduction of direct payments might not take into account the full costs of overheads and the responsibilities incurred by becoming an employer: 'If direct payments are going to be extended through legislation, then we have to make sure that they are not merely a back door way of reducing the cost of care' (quoted in Bond, 1996, p 20).

Since direct payments were formally implemented in April 1997, there has been ongoing concern about the hidden costs that managing payments may entail. In Scotland, many direct payment calculations did not appear to include National Insurance, sickness pay and contingency money (Witcher et al, 2000). In Staffordshire, a start-up payment of £25 to cover advertising costs, stationery, postage, telephone and travel expenses was welcomed by some recipients, but criticised by others as being inadequate:

> "An initial newspaper advert was placed and £25 did not cover the costs."

> "The money allowed for advertising needs to be reassessed. You cannot advertise in the local press for less than £80. Supermarkets often refuse to put in what they consider to be job applications on their advertising boards." (Leece, 2000, p 40)

Another key concern is the level of payments that local authorities choose to make. Since this sum is discretionary, it tends to vary considerably from area to area, and the amount of support that direct payment users receive is very much a 'postcode lottery'. In a Scottish study, hourly payments for PAs ranged from £3.60 to £11.64, and some authorities had no mechanisms for paying enhanced rates for unsocial hours or for workers with additional skills (Witcher et al, 2000). In 2007, Davey et al's (2007a) national survey provided one of the most detailed overviews of the current state of play. Although the picture that emerged was incredibly complicated, there was evidence to suggest that some local authorities may have been making insufficient payments and, in our view, setting direct payment recipients up to fail. While key findings are set out in Box 8.9, key areas for further analysis include significant variations across the UK, different levels of recognition of unsocial hours, the extent to which support services and start-up costs are fully funded and different approaches to dealing with any surpluses built up by direct payment recipients. Elsewhere, there is a tendency for eligibility criteria to get tighter and tighter, squeezing direct payment packages and allowing less and less time for specified activities (Hasler, 1999). Such tensions are also quickly picked up by front-line staff, who can sometimes feel trapped between the empowering rhetoric of direct payments and the severely financially constrained nature of current social care: "We're told one thing then another ... we're told there are no limits to direct payments, be creative one minute and told to watch our spending the next ... nobody knows what to expect" (Ellis, 2007, p 410).

Overall, NCIL's *Rough guide to managing personal assistants* (Vasey, 2000) is adamant that insufficient payments are a central obstacle to successful direct payment schemes:

> Some of the difficulties described in this book could be sorted out by a more substantial Direct Payment. Without enough money independent living becomes stressful and in some circumstances almost too stressful ... Money is one of the key factors in the crusade. It is both liberator and jailer and we have to resist all attempts to minimise care packages and maximise charging. If we fail then we will be in big trouble. We will have no money to pay for the other parts of our lives

(mortgages, children, vehicles) or to pay for the other mammoth costs associated with significant impairment. (Vasey, 2000, p 10)

Box 8.9: Direct payment rates

- Payment rates vary significantly across the UK, with Northern Ireland and Wales making lower payments than England and Scotland. However, rates can still vary even within regions.
- After deductions for tax and National Insurance, a direct payment recipient with a physical impairment can afford to pay on average £6.08 per hour.
- Different local authorities have different approaches to tax, National Insurance, holiday pay, sick pay, start-up costs, contingency funds and support costs.
- Most local authorities make direct payments at a rate lower than the average cost of preferred independent sector providers or of in-house domiciliary care.
- Some authorities pay a higher rate to service users who wish to use an agency.

(Davey et al, 2007a, ch 7)

A further financial difficulty concerns local authority monitoring processes. Throughout the campaign for direct payments, there was widespread concern about the financial implications of making payments to individual disabled people (see Chapter Three), and subsequent direct payment schemes have included clearly defined monitoring procedures to ensure that money is spent appropriately and efficiently. In many ways, this attention to financial detail is to be commended because it enables the local authority to audit its expenditure effectively, and protects disabled people against accusations of misusing their payments. However, there is also a danger that monitoring processes can become overly bureaucratic, acting as a disincentive to take up direct payments. To prevent this from happening, PSI/NCIL recommend that monitoring should be proportionate to the minimum requirements to protect the liabilities both of the disabled person and of the local authority (Hasler et al, 1998). This should include only setting up a separate bank account and providing copies of time sheets and bank statements – anything more may be considered excessive.

As a result, organisations like NCIL were initially critical of financial guidance issued by the Chartered Institute of Public Finance and Accountancy (CIPFA) (1998), which was deemed to be unnecessarily complex and obtrusive, failing to take account of the expertise of disabled people who had been running their own payment schemes for many years (NCIL, ndc; see also Box 8.10). While most disabled people want to demonstrate that they have spent their payments correctly, this must also be balanced against the underlying feeling that some direct payment recipients have that social services staff do not trust them and that they have to account to others for everything they do (Hasler, 1999; Maglajlic et al, 2000). This has since been clarified in subsequent CIPFA guidance, which is clear that 'monitoring arrangements should be light touch and proportionate to the level of risk involved' (CIPFA, 2007, p 17).

Box 8.10: CIPFA guidance

NCIL has great concerns over some of the guidance offered by CIPFA ... As this organisation's advice is viewed by [local authorities] as sacrosanct, any departure from their approach is met with almost total resistance. Direct Payment Support Schemes have contacted NCIL to complain that CIPFA monitoring and accounting arrangements are far too bureaucratic and complex for 'users' and social service practitioners to use practically on a day-to-day basis. The procedures are highly intrusive and burdensome, putting many people off the idea of managing a payment scheme ... Disabled people's established Independent Living Schemes have developed accounting and audit procedures for Direct or 'Third Party' Payments over a considerable number of years. They are therefore in a position to demonstrate highly 'workable' procedures which fully meet legal and public accountability requirements. Unfortunately CIPFA failed to involve such a body of expertise when they compiled their material.

(NCIL, ndd, p 5; for more recent CIPFA guidance with a very different approach, see CIPFA, 2007)

A final financial barrier is the tendency of some local authorities to impose cost ceilings on direct payment packages. Highlighted by organisations such as Age Concern (1998), NCIL (ndc) and Values Into Action (Holman and Bewley, 1999), the practice of limiting care packages through cost ceilings has been criticised by the government, who feel that this may result in premature admissions to residential care (DH, 1998b). Cost ceilings have also been opposed by a number of disability campaigners, who have argued that limiting the amount of community-based care available to disabled people contradicts the fundamental tenets of the Independent Living Movement:

> We do not support the use of cash ceilings, as we feel that they are entirely incompatible with needs led assessment. (NCIL, ndc, p 6)

> Many local authorities operate a cost ceiling as a way of controlling their community care budget. In some this is a guideline to care managers, in others it is a straightjacket. In authorities operating a rigid cost ceiling, people whose care needs exceed a set amount are directed to residential care ... People in residential care lead 'unnecessarily isolated and restricted lives'. They are unable to take paid work and, in all but a few cases, are unable to contribute to their local communities. Within the disability movement, campaigners have been arguing that it is both inefficient and inhumane to force people into residential care because of lack of funds for community-based support. The resulting

waste of human potential is a poor use of national resources, as well as personally damaging to the people concerned. (Hasler, 1997, p 13)

People generally want to live in their own homes if they can, and admission to institutional care ... can lead to lower self-confidence and a decline in activity. Yet the evidence is that many authorities are setting a financial ceiling on their domiciliary care packages, ... which can lead to premature admissions to care homes when care at home would have been more suitable. (DH, 1998b, p 14)

As Fernandez et al (2007, quoted in Hasler and Marshall, 2013, p 41) have argued:

The resource rationing process currently in place in local authorities, in the prevailing fiscal climate, could undermine options ... First, they affect care managers' abilities to offer Direct Payments at a sufficiently generous level, and hence their willingness to offer them at all. If the current regime is austere, local authorities are tending to respond by tightening eligibility criteria, which in turn means that only the most dependent people qualify for local authority support ... Second and relatedly, constraints on local budgets are perceived to limit the capacity to employ personal assistants appropriately.

Of course, these warnings came in 2007 – when the funding environment was relatively benign as compared to the current realities of local authority cuts. These are controversial issues that are beyond the scope of this book. However, the advent of personal budgets arguably makes some of this situation easier (while still not resolving all of the underlying issues). By linking financial resources to individual need in a more transparent way, personal budgets should spell out clearly what money is available for individuals to spend on their needs. While this does not get around the fact that there may not be enough money in the system as a whole, it gives the individual a sense of what they have available to meet their needs as best they can ('how much they have to play with', in everyday language). By being transparent about this, personal budgets also increase the opportunity for lobbying central government over funding levels or challenging local authority decisions. However, this is probably little consolation to someone in the here-and-now struggling to get their needs met in a system that most people think is dramatically under-funded (or to a worker trying to do their best without the resources to deliver). Thus, the risk remains that personalisation could become meaningless rhetoric (or, perhaps even worse, a smokescreen for further cuts) unless more fundamental change takes place.

Increasing inequity?

Of all the concerns that have been raised about direct payments and personal budgets, the perceived risk of increasing inequity and creating a 'two-tier' system has been one of the most prevalent and profound. If you asked many people working in public services what values they uphold, equity is likely to emerge as a defining feature of the welfare state – although many people would acknowledge that it is often difficult to achieve in practice. As Leece and Leece (2006, p 1380) suggest:

> It has been suggested ... that direct payments may be offered to and taken up disproportionately by well educated, more affluent, middle-class people, who are seen and feel able to take advantage of the opportunities offered by arranging their own support as opposed to accepting traditional service provision (Spandler, 2004; Leece, 2004). If this is the case, then the system of cash payments currently in place could be creating a two-tiered system of social support.

Certainly, some of the early history of direct payments can be interpreted in this way. As Leece and Leece point out, several early studies highlighted a significant number of direct payment recipients at local level who had prior experience of management roles and/or of supervising staff (Clark et al, 2004; Leece, 2004). Moreover, as Chapter Four has demonstrated, direct payments have been uneven in their spread, with certain regions and particular user groups benefiting more than others (see also Riddell et al, 2005). Given this, is there not a danger that direct payments might become the preserve only of the articulate and the rich (and even then, only in certain localities), leaving the less-well-off and the less-educated to directly provided services that have become even less responsive as a result of such 'cream-skimming'?

This is clearly a powerful argument and something to guard against at all costs. However, our view of the evidence to date is that this rests on a series of mistaken assumptions. As Le Grand (2007, pp 32–3) has pointed out, current services already favour the middle classes, who have always tended to benefit most from state welfare: 'the better off have louder voices: they also have better contacts and sharper elbows'. That this may be the case in social care too is suggested by a comparison of the cost of care packages versus level of need – in one case study local authority, funding under the traditional care management system was allocated very unevenly (with, for example, two people with similar needs receiving services costing £3,000 or £30,000 – see Duffy, 2008 for further discussion and analysis). In contrast, a system of personal budgets brings financial transparency to what was previously an opaque process – helping to ensure that people with equal needs start to receive equal resources. Rather than reducing equity, therefore, personal budgets may have the potential to increase it.

Turning to the specifics of direct payments and personal budgets, it is interesting to note that both have been criticised for benefiting different groups most. While direct payments have been taken up most enthusiastically by people with physical impairment, personal budgets developed out of the inclusion movement, and the majority of early budget holders were people with learning difficulties and their families (although, interestingly, the biggest user group is now older people). In one sense, this should be reassuring – given the very low base that learning disability services have come from historically, something that can work for people with learning difficulties (given the discrimination and low expectations they often face) ought potentially to work well for everyone.

When it comes to the more detailed research findings, Leece and Leece (2006) provide a fascinating overview based on an initial sample of 5,000 people who received a financial assessment from a case study local authority between 2002 and 2005. While their conclusions are inevitably tentative, they suggest that there were no statistically significant differences between direct payment recipients and users of traditional services in terms of wealth. Building on such findings, a 2008 review by the think-tank Demos (Leadbeater et al, 2008) addresses the issue of equity head on. For Demos, the assumption that personal budgets rely on a marketised form of social care that risks creating inequity is fundamentally misplaced for four main reasons:

- The current system does not treat people in a fair and consistent way, and there is often a poor fit between need and resources. At present, the system 'rewards the most articulate at the expense of the less confident: those who are most confident in complaining or most able to work the rules of the system stand more of a chance of getting the services they want. Giving people the same budgets to spend puts people on a much more equal footing' (pp 47–8).
- Personal budgets create a much fairer, more transparent link between need and resources.
- A key current inequity exists between those who can fund their own care and those who cannot. Thus, personal budgets 'offer state-funded clients the choices currently available only to the middle classes outside the system' (p 48).
- Personal budgets can work for all groups – including seldom-heard groups. By tailoring support to meet individual needs and aspirations, there is scope for self-directed support to be much more inclusive than previous ways of working. As an example, minority ethnic communities in Oldham make up 20% of the population, but only 1% of people accessing traditional social services. With the introduction of personal budgets, the figure rose close to 10% (p 48).

Finally, for all the concerns that have been raised about the longer-term implications of direct payments and personal budgets, the reality is that the solution to a potential 'two-tier system' is not to reduce everyone to the 'lower tier', but to work hard to make sure that everyone has access to the same opportunities for choice and control (that is, to achieve equity by raising standards to the highest level rather than by reducing them to the lowest common denominator). As Sapey and Pearson (2004, p 63) observe:

> How social workers act in relation to concerns about equity is an important indicator of attitude. If an improved or superior service via a direct payment is a sign of the success of the scheme, this should encourage social workers to view it positively rather than as a problem. A constructive response would be to promote the raising of standards of all services rather than criticise direct payments.

The exploitation of care workers and of women?

While there have been some changes over time, most personal care is provided by women (either as paid workers or as family carers), with the former often poorly paid, with poor career prospects and – in an age of zero-hours contracts – with increasingly uncertain job security. By definition, the advent of direct payments and personal budgets will therefore have a disproportionate impact on women, and any problems or shortcomings in new ways of working could easily lead to greater exploitation of women. A key contribution here comes from Ungerson (1997), who argues that direct payments may generate hardship for poorly paid women and other vulnerable groups. Rather than an internal market or quasi-market, Ungerson likens direct payments to a 'flea market' in which everyone involved is on a low income, the services delivered are not highly valued, some activity is illegal, and where it is possible, in some situations, to find a particular 'bargain' or 'treasure' who will work well beyond market and contractual requirements. Underlying this is a clear gender issue that Ungerson (1997, p 50) is quick to highlight:

> Although we know next to nothing about the kinds of people that work as personal assistants – except anecdotally – one can begin to guess who will come forward. Many of them will be women wishing to fit casual work, at unsociable hours, around the calls of their domestic lives and generate an income for themselves and their children. Some will be students in need of money to support their education, but [who] will be able to work in flexible packets of time. Others will be seeking housing solutions to their accommodation problems; some will be on benefit looking to enhance their incomes, either legally up to the earnings disregard for their particular benefit, or illegally beyond their benefit rules. Although direct payments will be 'monitored' by local authorities to ensure they are being spent properly on care services, there is nothing to suggest … that the market itself will be carefully policed. Hence, informal and illegal contractual arrangements, where the workers have no employment rights of any kind, are likely to develop.

Although Ungerson was writing before direct payments were formally implemented in April 1997, research findings do suggest that her concerns may have some weight. In 1993, a study of the experiences of disabled service users found that some payment recipients made cash-in-hand payments to PAs because of the inadequacy of the money they received (Morris, 1993a). Around the same time, Zarb and Nadash (1994) found that around 60% of respondents felt that the wages that they paid to PAs were too low. Many did not pay their workers holiday pay, and a few people made payments cash-in-hand. Should they receive any increase in funding, many people signalled their intention to increase their workers' wages and/or increase the number of hours worked. This led the researchers to the conclusion that 'although some people employing their own workers feel they have had to cut corners in the way they organise their support, this is invariably out of necessity rather than by choice' (Zarb and Nadash, 1994, p 42). Other studies have suggested that the rates of pay that direct payment recipients are able to offer do not reflect the types of work that PAs are expected to undertake, nor the skills that they may require (Glendinning et al, 2000a–c). Similar concerns have also been raised elsewhere in Europe, as a French director of social services has acknowledged: "Disabled people are happier and more independent [receiving direct payments], but the position of employees is fragile, with less training, less security and irregular hours of work" (quoted in Wellard, 1999, p 23).

More recently, Ungerson has developed her initial contribution with further research at a local level as well as cross-national research in five EU countries (see, for example, Ungerson, 1999, 2003, 2004, 2006; Ungerson and Yeandle, 2007). While this is detailed and important material, the essential argument is that changes in the boundary between work and care have resulted in new forms of relationship between disabled people, their families and employees – what is often called a 'commodification of care'. As a result, it is argued, direct employees often have less-clearly defined roles, which can lead to a decline in employee rights and working conditions, unregulated labour and difficulty for workers in leaving or exercising rights because of emotions such as guilt, friendship and feeling part of the family. Similar issues have also been raised by a range of other commentators, including some trade unions, who have voiced concerns about the potential for poor employment practices (see, for example, Lombard, 2008; see also Scourfield, 2005a for a broader discussion of possible workforce implications).

In response, disabled researchers such as Morris (1997) have emphasised that we should not be treating disabled people receiving direct payments any differently from other groups receiving state support. Thus, the majority of disabled employers probably do not pay cash-in-hand, and even those that do are probably no different from many non-disabled people who purchase services such as cleaning and childminding on an informal basis. In many ways, therefore, the receipt of direct payments is little different from the receipt of child benefit:

How many people pay someone to do their housework, and how many pay cash in hand? Those of us who do so may think of ourselves as good employers: we may pay at or above the local 'going rate', some of us may pay sick pay, bank holidays and holidays (I suspect more will not), but most of us don't deduct tax and national insurance or pay the employers' national insurance contribution. In fact, most of us would find it hard to get a cleaner if we insisted on anything other than a 'cash in hand' relationship. Does this mean that we are exploiting these low-paid women? ... The child benefit system is ... a system of cash payments made to individuals. I wonder how many mothers spend their child benefit in parts of the informal economy or on goods and services in the formal economy made or delivered by low-paid workers. Yet presumably Clare Ungerson would not wish to use this to question the value of the child benefit system. (Morris, 1997, pp 58–60)

For Morris, direct payments represent an opportunity to break down the stereotypes that disabled people have traditionally faced and establish their status as citizens, able to use cash payments in order to do what they want rather than what professional workers think they want. As a result, Morris feels that social researchers have a moral responsibility to collaborate with what she sees as a civil rights movement concerned with people's right to choice and control over their own lives. While both arguments (Morris's and Ungerson's) are persuasive, a way forward would surely seem to lie in the findings of Zarb and Nadash (1994): that many disabled people would want to pay higher wages if they received higher payments. Ultimately, the risk of exploiting women may lie not so much in the concept of direct payments itself, as in the way that many schemes are operationalised, restrictions on employing family members and the inadequate levels of payments that may sometimes be made.

More recently, a fascinating study commissioned by Skills for Care shed light on the employment conditions of PAs and the workforce implications of direct payments (IFF Research, 2008) – albeit these issues remain significantly under-researched (see, for example, Manthorpe et al, 2011a for research into the experience of people with learning difficulties). Based on interviews with 526 direct payment employers, a survey of 486 PAs and a more detailed telephone survey with 100 of the participating PAs, the study provides an important overview of a long-neglected issue. However, the results were controversial (see Box 8.11). As in previous studies, direct payment recipients reported high levels of satisfaction, and those with experience of directly provided services were clear that direct payments were superior. When the study was reported in the trade press, however, the focus tended to be on a small section of the report to do with training – only 7% of direct payment recipients had organised formal training for their staff, and this prompted debates about the extent to which disabled people were acting as good employers. What is staggering about the research, however, is the level of satisfaction reported by PAs. Overall, 95% of PAs were satisfied with their role (with only 1% quite unhappy and the rest neither happy nor unhappy), and 90% felt appreciated in their role either most of the time or frequently (IFF Research, 2008, pp 93–5). While these figures seem high for any job, they seem astounding in a role that is often low paid, unglamorous and emotionally and physically difficult. Moreover, on closer inspection, there are similar themes from other (albeit very small) studies – including some of Ungerson's own work, where some PAs express significant satisfaction with their work (see also Leece, 2006b). Overall, it appears as though PAs may have worse terms and conditions than local authority home carers, but may be happier, less stressed and attracted at least in part by the flexibility of the role. Quite how we have managed as a system to turn this into bad news is, at first glance, unclear. While these issues are likely to remain controversial, we believe that direct payments offer the possibility of a more satisfying, meaningful and productive relationship between the employee and their employer, and that this may be behind the high levels of satisfaction reported above. While this way of working does blur boundaries and may be problematic if things go wrong, it still seems to us to be much more positive than negative.

Box 8.11: The experience of employers and PAs

In 2008, a study of the workforce implications of direct payments found that:

- 79% of direct payment recipients were very satisfied with the support they were receiving, and 89% trust their PA completely. Both results compare very favourably to people's experiences of directly provided services, which were sometimes very negative.
- Direct payments were felt by the researchers to lead to better-quality and more reliable support, with fewer problems and fewer incidences of potential abuse than with direct services.
- Although being an employer was daunting for some, the majority did not feel like this (and people were happier with being an employer the longer they had been doing it, suggesting that experience can help to build confidence).
- Most people (66%) could find an appropriate PA quickly – but those who reported problems cited issues such as a low number of applicants, poor attitudes, not being willing to work the hours needed and/or not having the right personality.
- There are an estimated 76,000 people working as PAs in England, 87% of whom are women. One-third of PAs had no previous paid employment providing social care, so it seems likely that direct payments have encouraged a significant number of new people into the social care workforce.
- 95% of PAs were happy with their role and 90% felt appreciated most of the time or frequently. However, some were concerned about low pay (32%) and working more hours than they would ideally like (18%).

- Only 7% of employers had paid or arranged for training for PAs, although 19% provided training on the job themselves. The researchers concluded that some of this may be to do with a potential underfunding of direct payments, and many direct payment recipients were prepared to arrange training if this was properly funded.
- Direct payment recipients tended to emphasise personal factors (such as having a friendly attitude, being willing to work the hours required, adapting to the employer's individual needs and so on) more than previous skills and experience.
- 79% of employers would find a register of care workers useful, but only 46% thought it should be compulsory. When asked a second question, 71% would like to retain the right to employ someone not on the register. Among PAs, 87% thought registration was a good idea.

(IFF Research, 2008)

With the move to a new system of self-directed support, many of these issues are arguably easier to reconcile. In particular, there are two key issues:

- The initial resource allocation system developed by In Control provides something of a compromise. While the RAS did take the level of family support into account when allocating resources, it did not penalise people for having access to families in the same way as the old system. Thus, someone without any family support would get more resources than someone with the same needs and plenty of family support – but the latter would still be entitled to more assistance than they might have been under current eligibility criteria. As personal budgets are rolled out there are different approaches to RAS in different places, but it remains perfectly possible to build assumptions about the availability of family support into the model. Thus, if we decided as a society that someone with access to family support should have exactly the same support as someone without access, we could design a RAS accordingly. Equally, we could weight the RAS so that someone without any other support received more. Essentially, a 'RAS' is merely a process; while it cannot resolve underlying tensions about the role of women in our society, we could use it to implement the results of any more profound debate we wanted to have on these issues.
- By being informed how much money is available to meet their needs, the individual can now decide how they want this money spent on their behalf, whether it be via private/voluntary/public services, via friends and family and/ or via something that does not look like 'services' or 'support' at all. While this does not totally remove some of the issues described above, it gives individuals and families much more space to decide upon the types of relationship they want to have with each other (and leaves social care workers and the state out of this complex and sensitive territory). Although social workers still have a role to play in ensuring needs are met and in ensuring people are safe in situations where adult protection concerns apply, the move to personal budgets seems to simplify much of the previous debate by leaving much more to individual choice, preference and circumstances.

What long-term impact personal budgets may have on the social work workforce is unclear – but early insights from the initial government individual budgets pilots suggest that stress initially increased significantly, with new processes and initiatives leaving workers feeling even more burdened and that they had even less discretion than before (Wilberforce et al, 2014; see also Slasberg et al, 2012a for discussion of the way in which some local authorities have tended to respond to personal budgets by adding extra processes and bureaucracy). Whether this is a product of personal budgets per se, or more to do with poor implementation or the danger of pilots increasing work by overlaying new approaches on top of previous systems remains to be seen. As Wilberforce et al (2014, p 827) observe:

> The ever-evolving nature of social work in England will continue to be a subject of great interest, particularly where the content of such work contributes to high levels of stress amongst its practitioners ... This paper has demonstrated its utility and its potential for investigating the impact of any number of legislative, policy, organisational or practice changes on the job characteristics of social workers. The findings of this paper indicate that the IB pilots may have had a detrimental impact on the risk of stress, and this is supported by qualitative interviews with staff, but these also suggested that some pressures may reduce as the policy becomes established. Further research is warranted to investigate the impact of the national Personal Budget roll-out, especially in the context of a new service climate characterised by financial austerity and organisational upheaval.

Risk

As pressure for direct payments mounted, a key feature of the government's initial refusal to implement such a scheme was the argument that making cash payments to disabled service users would leave them at risk. This was rejected by disabled campaigners (who argued that they were already at risk from substandard local authority services), and ultimately defeated. However, even after the successful implementation of direct payments, concerns about risk have continued to surface (Burrows, 2001; George, 2001) and do raise doubts about direct payments as currently conceptualised.

In most of the early literature, the issue of risk was either downplayed or rejected outright. In a Department of Health (1998a) promotional video, one commentator is adamant that the risk associated with direct payments is minimal and that taking risks is a central feature of being in control of one's own services. A similar argument is also put forward by NCIL, who emphasise that taking risks is an important citizen right and that the empowerment offered by direct payments can actually reduce risks by making people more in control of their lives:

> Protection from abuse is linked to empowerment in that it is the common experience of disabled people that the more we are in control of our lives, and the support we need to lead them, the less likely we are to find ourselves in abusive situations. It must be recognised that historically, disabled people's freedom of movement, choice and control has been regularly denied or curtailed in the name of 'safety' ... Disabled people must be given the same rights to take risks as all citizens. (NCIL, 1999, pp 4, 8)

Elsewhere, there is evidence to suggest that some local authorities have responded to perceived risk by adopting very strict and rigid policies that deter potential direct payment recipients and undermine the flexibility that this way of working is meant to deliver (see, for example, CSCI, 2004; Hasler and Marshall, 2013). This seems to be particularly the case when designing audit and reporting processes, which can sometimes be over-prescriptive and disproportionate to risk (CSCI, 2004). As one person remarked in Henwood and Hudson's (2007b, p 51) study: "we don't worry about all the money we waste on crap institutional provision, but yet we will worry about giving someone £20!"

However, the fact remains that people working in adult social care are tasked with considering issues of risk – and that we live in a very risk-averse culture where policy makers and the media can be extremely critical of local authorities if things are perceived to 'go wrong'. With the advent of personal budgets, some people felt that these issues would recede, as there would be a spectrum of options available to people about what control they wanted to have over the money itself (which could include council-managed budgets). There was also initial optimism that the concepts underpinning personal budgets could begin to challenge traditional assumptions and help promote a more positive risk-enabling culture. As we suggested in our second edition, one of the limitations of the previous system is that it assumes that most people are either untrustworthy or incapable, and thus is overly bureaucratic and cumbersome. By shifting to a system where we assume that most people are capable and can be trusted, we are then able to focus scarce resources on the small number of cases where this may not be true (for example, where there are concerns about adult protection). By supporting people to exercise greater choice and control, we arguably put them at less risk of abuse – because they are more confident, have more community links and are better able to recognise and respond to potential abuse when it occurs.

In practice, these debates have not gone away – despite evidence to suggest that there do not seem to be higher levels of safeguarding referrals for people receiving council-managed personal budgets or direct payments, as compared to all social care users, and that 'some of the fears expressed by practitioners and managers may have been overstated' (Stevens et al, 2014, p 4). Early on, it seemed as though those leading local safeguarding processes had not been adequately involved in debates about personalisation (see, for example, Glendinning et al, 2008; Manthorpe et al, 2009b, 2011b), albeit more recent research suggests that there has been a degree of progress over time (Manthorpe et al, 2015b). We suspect that these debates may never be fully resolved, but our own view was summarised in a paper on risk and regulation for the JRF (Glasby, 2012b; see Box 8.12). In the mean time, risk is likely to remain a key element of social care policy and practice – and front-line workers and the services within which they work will face a dilemma about the balance to be struck between risk aversion and risk enablement (see Carr, 2010, 2011 for further discussion).

Box 8.12 Whose risk is it anyway?

The advent of personalisation raises a series of issues about risk and regulation – with increasingly polarised views. While some believe that direct payments and personal budgets could put people more at risk of abuse and exploitation, others feel that they may reduce risk by giving people greater control over their lives. Against this background, this paper argues that:

- Risk is important – but people using services often perceive this in a disempowering way as something that is imposed on them by the system.
- We make people safe not by segregating them, but by building their confidence and by more fully connecting them to their communities.
- We reduce risks if we identify them in advance and plan what to do in an emergency – and the support planning involved in personal budgets can help to improve this.
- We might protect people better if we could focus our safeguards on those people who really need it – rather than spreading our resources too thin by trying to put everyone through the same system (which can be unnecessary for some and not enough for others).
- Personalisation and safeguarding are (or at least should be) two sides of the same coin – although they are too often seen as separate processes locally.
- Adequate support is crucial and this must be fully tailored to the individual.

Overall, key messages for policy and practice are that:

1. Risk should be shared between the person who takes the risk and the system that is trying to support them.
2. Personal budgets and direct payments are not a panacea, and abuse and exploitation will still exist in an era of personalisation. Despite this, the different options available via self-directed support may give workers more of spectrum of options and different ways of responding.
3. Our approaches need to be proportionate to risk – but we often subject new ways of working to greater scrutiny than previous approaches.
4. Similarly, regulation needs to be proportionate to risk – and people's willingness and readiness to take positive risks will vary according to individual context. We therefore need a system of regulation that can be as personalised as the services we are now seeking to provide.

5. The current financial context could place people at risk by reducing access to practical and peer support, contingency funds and the availability of experienced professional staff when needed. While personalisation may help us to spend the money we have as well as we can, we have to invest to save – and some of the cuts that may be implemented in the coming months and years could prove false economy if they prevent personalisation from flourishing.

6. The biggest risk in the current financial and policy context is that we scrutinise and regulate personalisation to death, paying lip-service to it but killing any scope for genuine creativity and gradually allowing the old system to recreate itself under the new language. This seems the worst of all worlds and something to be actively avoided.

(Glasby, 2011, pp 4–5; see also Littlechild et al, 2011; Glasby, 2012b)

Practical challenges and support mechanisms

Managing direct payments is not easy, and recipients choosing to employ their own PAs face a series of practical challenges to overcome, including recruiting and retaining good staff, being a good employer, handling tax and National Insurance and accounting for funds received. Although many of these issues are dealt with in much greater detail in the practical resources listed at the end of this chapter, it is important that service users and their social workers are aware of the practical challenges that direct payments can raise and are clear about the way in which these challenges are to be overcome. Unless these issues are carefully considered, the result can be a situation in which service users unused to managing their own payments may be left to struggle on alone, without adequate support. At best, this will be stressful for the individuals concerned and may prejudice them against direct payments in the future. At worst, it could lead to a breakdown in care arrangements, with potential financial and legal implications for the service user and/or the local authority. Certainly the alleged complexity of direct payments is something that some people (particularly, the evidence suggests, older people and people with mental health problems) may find daunting – at least at first. Managing a payment and (possibly) employing staff are new skills for many people, and most of us would need significant information, training and support to take on these roles. While some studies suggest that such complexity can be perceived as a barrier (see, for example, Help the Aged, 2002; Ridley and Jones, 2003; CSCI, 2004), others argue that people are put off by difficulties in accessing direct payments – not a lack of desire to try this way of working (see, for example, Stainton and Boyce, 2004). Moreover, there is also evidence to suggest that many people do not perceive direct payments to be overly daunting, particularly when they have had a chance to build their confidence over time (see, for example, IFF Research, 2008). Overall, there are two key ways in which the perceived complexity of direct payments can be reduced:

- Local authorities should ensure that the procedures they put in place are no more onerous than is absolutely essential. In some areas, direct payments seem so difficult and bureaucratic to access that numbers of recipients remain low. While this may be to do with the culture of individual local authorities, it can sometimes be the result of a deliberate attempt to pay lip-service to the concept of direct payments while also restricting access.
- The success of direct payments depends significantly on access to support – particularly peer support (see below for further discussion).

Throughout the literature, the need for adequate support structures is an almost constant theme (see, for example, Simpson with Campbell, 1996; Dunnicliff, 1999; Hasler et al, 1999; Dawson, 2000; Glendinning et al, 2000c; Leece, 2000), and the absence of such support can be a major barrier that is difficult to overcome (Witcher et al, 2000). This was recognised by the Department of Health (1997, 2000) from the very beginning, and has also been highlighted through evaluations undertaken by the Social Services Inspectorate (Fruin, 2000, p 16). In six authorities where direct payments were in place, users were found to need assistance in starting to receive payments and managing them on an ongoing basis, in terms of both administrative issues and psychological support. This was sometimes provided by a local disability organisation, by other voluntary agencies or by specialist social services staff, although there was no evidence of peer support or self-help groups in any of the authorities concerned. However, nowhere is the importance of adequate support more apparent than in PSI/ NCIL guidance for local authorities seeking to implement and manage direct payment schemes (Hasler et al, 1999). To emphasise the centrality of effective support mechanisms, the guidance notes that, in areas where disabled people are successfully managing direct payments, there is nearly always an established support service to assist them:

> Support services are perhaps the most fundamental part of a successful direct payments scheme. The purpose of direct payments support services is to ensure that adequate advice, information and support are available to disabled people so that they may feel confident to undertake the complexities of using direct payments to employ and manage their own staff. Such support also ensures that individuals using a direct payment are operating legally and efficiently. The support service has to be properly funded and responsive. (Hasler et al, 1999, p 11)

After the Community Care (Direct Payments) Act came into force in 1997, more and more schemes have developed, often provided by Centres for Independent Living, and disabled people have proved extremely capable of rising to the practical issues that direct payments present. Although managing direct payments may be difficult at times, this should not stop disabled people from attempting to do so.

Above all, this is the resounding message that emerges from NCIL's *Rough guide to managing personal assistants*:

> Direct Payments really represent a golden opportunity for disabled people. They are the means by which we close the chapter of disability history called 'Institutions' and move on to the part of the story where we get a crack at living just like everybody else. With the right facilitation any disabled person, whatever their impairment, can take control and be free to get on with life. It all seems so simple, but of course like so many things it is just a bit more complicated than it first appears … We are all wrestling with the same issues. Everybody finds it an effort, at least some of the time, because it is basically management work that we are involved in here and management is rarely easy. In business, managers are paid large sums and then often do it badly. We get paid nothing and cannot afford to fail, not only because our living arrangements will instantly be in tatters, but because there is a view widely held by the powers that be that we are not up to the job. This book [The rough guide] is a celebration of disabled people's undoubted ability to get on with a difficult job in order to get a life. (Vasey, 2000, pp 7–8)

Although they may have different names, all support services should include four core features:

- peer support (so that disabled people can share information and experiences, develop practical solutions to problems and support each other);
- information (covering all aspects of independent living and direct payments, available in a range of formats and languages);
- advice and/or advocacy (to assist disabled people to manage their payments and find solutions to any problems);
- training (about independent living, recruiting staff, time management, building relationships with staff, legal responsibilities and administrative duties) (Hasler et al, 1999, pp 12–15).

In addition to this, some support schemes may offer a payroll service, employ staff on behalf of the service user and hold registers of PAs (see Hasler and Marshall, 2013 for some practical examples of the support available – and of existing PA registers). However, there has been ongoing evidence to suggest that some direct payment recipients may not always receive the practical support they need (Davey et al, 2007a), and that many user-led Centres for Independent Living may be finding it difficult to provide the levels of support they would like (Barnes and Mercer, 2006). Despite a number of national pledges, this has only got worse in recent years, with a difficult financial environment bringing challenges for user-led organisations as well as the local authorities that contract with them. This is deeply to be regretted, as all the available evidence suggests that user-led organisations and peer support are particularly powerful and helpful ways of supporting people who are considering direct payments (Hasler and Marshall, 2013).

With the advent of personal budgets, the need for support probably becomes more straightforward and more complex at the same time (if that is possible). With everyone receiving a personal budget able to play a greater role in planning their support, there is now a much broader range of choices with regard to how much control people want over the resources that are available to meet their needs (see Chapter Five for more detailed discussion). For those who want to control how their needs are met, but do not want to manage the practicalities of this themselves, the concept of self-directed support offers a new and exciting way forward. Of course, within this there will still be many people who want to receive at least part of their personal budget in the form of a direct payment – and these people in particular will need access to the same practical support as in the early days of direct payments. However, a system of self-directed support seems to point to a potential future where there is a much broader range of options available locally, and where people can choose which sort of support will be best for them – whether this be from a social worker, a family member, a service provider, a broker, a high street solicitor, a Centre for Independent Living or another source altogether. To us, this is both exciting and potentially liberating (for staff and service users alike), but also daunting – if the history of direct payments tells us just one thing, it is that failure to ensure that adequate support is available can set people up to fail and be a way of undermining the very choice and control that should be at the heart of this way of working. Hand in hand with access to meaningful support must also go active attempts to simplify the current system and make it as accessible and as proportionate to risk as possible – and recent experience suggests that this may remain a challenge.

SUMMARY

Despite the positives emphasised in Chapter Seven, direct payments and personal budgets (as currently conceived) may also bring a number of disadvantages that need to be acknowledged and overcome. Introduced by a Conservative government committed to rolling back the frontiers of the welfare state, there is a potential contradiction between the emphasis of the Independent Living Movement on choice and control, and an initial (and perhaps ongoing?) government agenda influenced by flawed notions of consumerism. Implemented against the backdrop of attempts to curtail public expenditure, direct payment schemes may not have received sufficient funding, resulting in financial difficulties for some local authorities, inadequate payments and support arrangements, low wages for PAs and the potential exploitation of women. Following the advent of personal budgets, moreover, other difficulties have included the need to balance empowerment against risk and the perceived danger that these ways of working may exacerbate existing inequalities. With public spending once again being significantly curtailed, some previous gains may now be under threat – and there remains a risk that personalisation could be exploited by government as a means of making ideologically motivated cuts in public services seem slightly less unpalatable. Throughout, though, a key barrier has been the attitude and practices of front-line social workers, who occupy an important gatekeeping role and can sometimes hinder rather than facilitate the dissemination of information about direct payments and personal budgets. Thus, whatever is happening in terms of government priorities, it will be workers at local level who are responsible for delivering national policy and who have a key role to play in making sure we implement direct payments and personal budgets in a way that is consistent with the principles of independent living, citizenship and equity.

IMPLICATIONS FOR POLICY AND PRACTICE

- Direct payments and personal budgets can appeal across the political spectrum, and there is some evidence to suggest that different groups may promote these ways of working for different reasons. In the short term, this has built momentum for change; in the longer term it could lead to tensions if the interests of the different groups diverge.
- Front-line workers have a key role to play in the development of direct payments/personal budgets – either in promoting these ways of working or in restricting access.
- Calculating the appropriate level of direct payments is crucial if people are to be able to meet their needs and to be good employers. Making inadequate payments sets people up to fail.
- Direct payments and personal budgets change the nature of the relationship between the disabled person and the workers who may meet their needs (in a way that can be liberating but which is also contentious).
- Risk is a key element of social care, and debates continue as to whether direct payments and personal budgets reduce or increase risk.
- Direct payments in particular have a series of practical implications in terms of managing and administering resources. This can become a barrier to access if systems are unnecessarily restrictive/onerous or if appropriate support is not available.
- Linked to this, access to practical support (especially peer support) is a crucial component of the success of many direct payment schemes. This is also true of personal budgets, although self-directed support arguably allows the individual to choose from a broader range of support mechanisms.

RECOMMENDED READING AND USEFUL WEBSITES

Of all the critiques of direct payments and the discussions of differences between civil rights and consumerist approaches, Spandler's (2004) review provides a helpful summary. For more general discussion of issues to do with rights, empowerment and consumerism, a range of different views and contributions are provided by Ellis (2005), Ferguson (2007), Rummery (2006), Sapey and Pearson (2004), Stainton (2002, 2005), Riddell et al (2005) and Scourfield (2007).

A series of critical essays on personalisation more generally is found in Beresford's (2014b) short book, *Personalisation*.

Ellis's (2007) study of front-line assessment and care management practice provides a fascinating insight into the pressures practitioners face, the way they ration access to direct payments and the justifications they put forward to legitimise this practice. Simon Duffy's (2007) paper on 'Care management and self-directed support' is a concise and helpful summary of the implications of personal budgets for care management and professional social work.

For a discussion of the financial implications of direct payments/personal budgets, see the Audit Commission (2006) and Duffy and Waters' (2008) 'The economics of self-directed support', as well as national evaluations by Glendinning et al (2008) and Forder et al (2012). For a critique of some of this evidence, see Slasberg et al (2012a–b; 2014).

For discussions on the social care workforce, see the initial debate between Jenny Morris (1997) and Clare Ungerson (1997). Other sources include:

- ongoing research into this topic by Ungerson (1999, 2003, 2004, 2006; Ungerson and Yeandle, 2007);
- a study on the workforce implications of direct payments commissioned by Skills for Care (IFF Research, 2008);
- a Department of Health (2011b) framework for supporting PAs;
- a SCIE (2012) briefing for PAs;
- Skills for Care (2011, 2012) research into the factors disabled people feel are important in their relationship with PAs, together with subsequent practical guidance. Skills for Care has also produced a toolkit to support people employing PAs (www.skillsforcare.org.uk/employingpas);
- critical reflections on recent policy from UNISON (Pile, 2014).

For an early review of the evidence around risk and personalisation, see Carr's (2010) review for SCIE or Glasby's (2011) more provocative scoping paper for the JRF (see also ongoing research by Manthorpe et al, 2009b, 2010, 2015b; Manthorpe and Samsi, 2013 for developments over time).

For a national overview of the state of play with regard to the provision of support services, see Barnes and Mercer's (2006) *Independent futures* and Davey et al's (2007a) survey of direct payment support schemes. Good practice examples are also provided in the review by Hasler and Marshall (2013). Sources of practical support include local Centres of Independent Living and other user-led organisations. At a national level, Disability Rights UK (www.disabilityrightsuk.org) was formed in 2012 from a merger of RADAR, the Disability Alliance and NCIL, and its website provides a series of factsheets, policy briefings and campaign updates.

REFLECTIVE EXERCISES

1. Re-read the key social care policy documents that commit to a policy of direct payments and personal budgets (see Chapters Three and Five) – to what extent do these reflect a consumer model and to what extent do they reflect a commitment to citizenship? Do they sometimes do both at the same time? What words are used to justify these policies, and does the reality of the policy commitment match the rhetoric of the policy document? What can you do to make sure that these ways of working remain true to the underlying values of the independent living movement?

2. For readers in practitioner roles, what are your personal views about direct payments and personal budgets – and to what extent do these shape how you give information and how you work with others? What role are you playing in opening up or closing down choice?

3. How are direct payment rates and personal budgets calculated locally? How easy is it to find this information, and how transparent are funding levels? How do these compare to the cost of directly provided services?

4. Do you know or can you find out who receives a direct payment and a personal budget locally? Do some groups benefit more than others? What can you do to promote these options to everyone, irrespective of their background?

5. What impact are direct payments and personal budgets having on the social care workforce? Will they lead to better relationships between employers and PAs, or could they lead to the exploitation of workers? What do you or your local authority know about people working as PAs locally, why they choose to do this role and what their experiences are? What experience do disabled employers have of recruiting and managing their own staff? In addition, what impact are personal budgets having on the social work workforce? Where there are potential negatives, are these to do with the transition to new approaches – or are there more fundamental barriers? What can the social work profession as a whole do to maximise the potential advantages and minimise potential limitations?

6. Write a list of the potential benefits of direct payments/personal budgets and some of the potential risks. How do the two lists compare? Reflecting on your own life, what risks do you take as part of leading an everyday life – and how would you feel about the balance between risk enablement and risk aversion if you were using services?

7. Reflecting on some of the practicalities of direct payments and personal budgets, do you know what practical and peer support exists locally? Talk to someone receiving a personal budget and/or a direct payment – how supported did they feel when making decisions about their care and when managing the subsequent practicalities? Where people have experience of different types of support, what were the pros and cons of each?

NINE

Conclusion – implications for community care

At their best, direct payments and personal budgets have the capacity to transform the lives of disabled people and to enrich the jobs of social care staff. Implemented after a sustained campaign by disabled people's organisations, direct payments are potentially revolutionary in terms of the opportunities they offer to enhance the choice, control, health and well-being of previously marginalised groups of disabled people. In some local authorities, direct payments have been implemented with enthusiasm, benefitting service users, improving satisfaction with care arrangements and leading to greater cost-efficiency. However, this has not always been the case, and some local authorities were slow to recognise and capitalise on the advantages that direct payments offer. Often, patterns of implementation have been strongly affected by regional variations, with particular areas of the country dragging their heels and hindering progress. Early on, in particular, little consideration seemed to have been given to the needs of user groups other than people with physical impairments; and access to payments was often denied to certain categories of people altogether (despite government guidance). While this was partly due to the initial wording and focus of legislation and official documentation, it was also the result of discriminatory attitudes and a failure to provide appropriate and accessible information to a range of user groups. Although their contribution was and continues to be significant, the fact remains that direct payments often felt like something bolted on to the current system and their capacity to transform the system as a whole was too often constrained.

More recently, the development of personal budgets has sought to build on what was good about direct payments in order to create a new system of social care. Perhaps unsurprisingly, this has been more difficult and more contested than might have first appeared – and some of the early optimism in our second edition has given way to a more cautious response in an era of austerity. While there remain significant potential positives, there are also risks that personal budgets will be implemented badly in some areas, that the language of personalisation may be co-opted for less-than-empowering ends and that the in-built ability of systems to resist change may stifle innovation and creativity. As we have argued throughout, perhaps the role of practitioners in such a situation is to acquaint themselves with the facts and the key debates, decide what they think and find ways of building on the positives and limiting the potential negatives. For Hasler and Marshall (2013, p 25):

> The conclusion… is that we do know what works – what is lacking is the will to apply what we know. The basic elements enabling successful

171

take-up of direct payments have not changed: the biggest barriers to getting these lessons applied appear to be a culture of risk aversion and a failure to trust both user-led support and user-directed solutions. The essential elements of making personal budgets succeed are also the things that will support more take-up of direct payments. Attempting to impose limits and tight controls on personal budgets will reduce their usefulness. The essential values of personalisation are the same as the essential values of independent living, which was the starting point for direct payments. So, the route to successfully increasing the take-up of direct payments is to embrace the values of personalisation, to take a creative and whole-hearted approach to personal budgets and to support the wider range of third sector and community-led support systems that enable successful management of direct payments.

Implications for practice

The attitude of front-line workers is crucial to the success or failure of direct payments and personal budgets. Disabled people often currently rely on social workers and care staff for a great deal of information and cannot be expected to make informed choices without accurate and accessible advice about the options available to them. Evidence to date suggests that social workers play an important gatekeeping role, and that those people who receive direct payments/personal budgets often do so at least in part because of information and support provided by a social worker. At the same time, research also suggests that some practitioners may be relatively uninformed about direct payments and personal budgets and/or suspicious about the implications for their work. In many cases, fears about an erosion of public services, about losing power and status, about workload implications, and about the dangers of creating demands that cannot be met, may be hindering the progress of direct payments and personal budgets. In this scenario, it is not disabled people making informed decisions to reject new ways of working, but their social workers effectively depriving them of access to direct payments and personal budgets by failing to provide support and information. If direct payments and personal budgets really are to become a central feature of mainstream social care, there needs to be much greater emphasis on training for front-line workers and on the provision of accessible information. Although we hope that this book goes some way towards promoting the concepts of direct payments and personal budgets, much more work will be required by social work trainers and educators to ensure that staff are appropriately trained, informed and have the right value base for the job they occupy. It will then be down to individual workers to ensure that the people with whom they work:

- are fully informed about the options available to them;
- have the opportunity to think and talk through the advantages and disadvantages of direct payments and personal budgets;

- have sufficient time to make a decision about the type of support they would like to receive;
- have access to peer support so that they can benefit from the experiences of other disabled people.

Overall, despite all the complexities, it is our firm belief that direct payments/personal budgets offer practitioners a new and extremely exciting way of working, empowering service users to be more in control of their own lives. If we get this right, this could be a way of helping workers to reconnect to the value base of the profession, and could free up scarce resources to focus on those most in need of support. If we don't get this right, then everyone will suffer – and there remains much to play for.

Implications for policy

In addition to changes in the training and attitudes of front-line workers, a number of policy measures will be required to promote direct payments and personal budgets, removing existing limitations while at the same time retaining the many advantages that these ways of working have to offer. Throughout, the key test will be the extent to which the system as a whole can hold on to the underlying value bases of direct payments and personal budgets, allowing them to remain sufficiently flexible to be effective and preventing the old system from reinventing itself. Ironically, neither direct payments nor personal budgets were at their most vulnerable when they began in humble circumstances as good ideas for future policy and practice, and started to spread from the bottom up. Instead, the biggest risk comes now that both are central features of national policy, and there seems a real danger that either/both could become incorporated into mainstream practice but get watered down to such an extent that they lose most of their power and potential impact. As Dowson (2002, p 57, quoted in Spandler and Vick, 2006, p 113) has previously warned: 'Little by little, the necessary ingredients of IF [independent funding] will be omitted, weakened, re-defined, downgraded; until IF has become something that no longer poses a threat to the system.'

The history of community care is full of new developments that promised much during pilots, but failed to deliver because of the way in which they were implemented. The challenge for policy makers, managers, practitioners, service users and students alike is now to make sure that this does not happen again. In particular, both direct payments and personal budgets could easily be a tool to accelerate consumerist reforms of public services, disguise draconian cuts and pass off state responsibilities to individuals struggling to overcome reductions and cuts in a wide range of services. Equally, they could be a powerful mechanism for promoting citizenship, civil rights, independent living, choice and control. Ultimately, policy makers and local leaders will need to be clear about which of these goals they are pursuing so that everyone else knows where they stand.

References

6, P. (2003) 'Giving consumers of British public services more choice: what can be learned from recent history?', *Journal of Social Policy*, vol 32, no 2, pp 239–70.

Abbott, D. (2003) *Direct payments for young disabled people*, York: Joseph Rowntree Foundation (JRF).

ADASS (Association of Directors of Adult Social Services) (2014) *ADASS personalisation survey 2014: national overview report*, available online via www.adass.org.uk/PersonalisationSurvey2014/Report/ (accessed 22/05/2015).

Adams, I. (1998) *Ideology and politics in Britain today*, Manchester: Manchester University Press.

Age Concern (1998) 'Extend direct payments to over 65s', *Care Plan*, vol 5, no 2, pp 14–16.

Age Concern (2000) *Direct payments from social services*, Factsheet 24, London: Age Concern England.

Age UK (2010) *Personalisation in practice: lessons from experience – making personal budgets, support planning and brokerage work for older people in later life*, London: Age UK.

Alakeson, V. (2007) *The case for extending self-direction in the NHS*, London: Social Market Foundation.

Alakeson, V. (2010a) *International developments in self-directed care*, New York: The Commonwealth Fund.

Alakeson, V. (2010b) *Active patient: the case for self-direction in healthcare*, Sheffield/Birmingham: Centre for Welfare Reform/Health Services Management Centre.

Alakeson, V. (2014) *Delivering personal health budgets: a guide to policy and practice*, Bristol: The Policy Press.

Alakeson, V. and Perkins, R. (2012) *Recovery, personalisation and personal budgets*, London: Centre for Mental Health/NHS Confederation.

Alcock, P. (1996) *Social policy in Britain: themes and issues*, Basingstoke: Macmillan.

Alzheimer's Society (2011) *Getting personal? Making personal budgets work for people with dementia*, London: Alzheimer's Society.

Andrisani, P. and Nestel, G. (1976) 'Internal–external control as contributor to and outcome of work experience', *Journal of Applied Psychology*, vol 61, no 2, pp 156–65.

Arksey, H. and Baxter, K. (2012) 'Exploring the temporal aspects of direct payments', *British Journal of Social Work*, vol 42, no 1, pp 147–64.

Askheim, O.P. (2003) 'Empowerment as guidance for professional social work: an act of balancing on a slack rope', *European Journal of Social Work*, vol 6, no 3, pp 229–40.

Audit Commission (1986) *Making a reality of community care*, London: HMSO.

Audit Commission (1992) *Community care: managing the cascade of change*, London: HMSO.

Audit Commission (2006) *Choosing well: analysing the costs and benefits of choice in local public services*, London: Audit Commission.

Audit Commission (2010) *Financial management of personal budgets: challenges and opportunities for councils*, London: Audit Commission.

Auld, F. (1999) *Community Care (Direct Payments) Act 1996: analysis of responses to local authority questionnaire on implementation – England*, London: DH.

Barnes, C. (1995) *From national to local: an evaluation of the effectiveness of national disablement information providers' information services to local disablement information providers*, London: British Council of Disabled People.

Barnes, C. (1997) *Older people's perceptions of direct payments and self-operated support schemes*, Leeds: British Council of Disabled People Research Unit.

Barnes, C. and Mercer, G. (2006) *Independent futures: creating user-led disability services in a disabling society*, Bristol: The Policy Press.

Barnes, M. (1997) *Care, communities and citizens*, London: Longman.

Barnes, M. and Walker, A. (1996) 'Consumerism versus empowerment: a principled approach to the involvement of older service users', *Policy & Politics*, vol 24, no 4, pp 375–94.

Barnett, H. (1918) *Canon Barnett: his life, work and friends – volume one*, London: John Murray.

Barret, G. and Hudson, M. (1997) 'Changes in district nursing workload', *Journal of Community Nursing*, vol 11, no 3, pp 4–8.

Baxter, K. et al (2008) *Domiciliary care agency responses to increased user choice*, York: Social Policy Research Unit.

Baxter, K. et al (2013) 'Managed personal budgets for older people: what are English local authorities doing to facilitate personalized and flexible care?', *Public Money & Management*, vol 33, no 6, pp 399–406.

Beardshaw, V. (1988) *Last on the list: community services for people with physical disabilities*, London: King's Fund.

Becker, S. (1997) *Responding to poverty: the politics of cash and care*, Basingstoke: Macmillan.

Bennett, S. (2008) *Commissioning for personalisation: a framework for local authority commissioners*, London: DH.

Beresford, P. (1996) 'Meet the diversity of need', *Care Plan*, vol 2, no 4, p 14.

Beresford, P. (2011/12) 'Are personal budgets necessarily empowering for service users? If not, what's it all about?', *Research, Policy and Planning*, vol 29, no 1, pp 37–43.

Beresford, P. (2014a) 'Advancing the positives of personalisation/person-centred support: a multi-perspective view', in C. Needham and J. Glasby (eds) *Debates in personalisation*, Bristol: The Policy Press.

Beresford, P. (2014b) *Personalisation*, Bristol: The Policy Press.

Beresford, P. et al (2005) *Developing social care: service users' vision for adult support*, London: Social Care Institute for Excellence.

Bewley, C. (1998) *Choice and control: decision-making and people with learning difficulties*, London: Values Into Action.

Bewley, C. (2000) 'Care managers can be champions for direct payments', *Care Plan*, vol 6, no 4, pp 13–16.

Bewley, C. and McCulloch, L. (2004) *Helping ourselves: direct payments and the development of peer support*, York: JRF.

Bignall, T. and Butt, J. (2000) *Between ambition and achievement: young black disabled people's views and experiences of independence and independent living*, Bristol/York: The Policy Press/JRF.

Blackender, L. and Prestidge, J. (2014) 'Pan-London personalised budgets for rough sleepers', *Journal of Integrated Care*, vol 22, no 1, pp 23–26.

Blyth, C. and Gardner, A. (2007) '"We're not asking for anything special": direct payments and the carers of disabled children', *Disability and Society*, vol 22, no 3, pp 235–49.

Bond, H. (1996) 'State of independence', *Community Care*, 4–10 April, pp 20–1.

Bosanquet, H. (1914) *Social work in London 1869–1912: a history of the Charity Organisation Society*, London: John Murray.

Brandon, D., Maglajlic, R. and Given, D. (2000) 'The information deficit hinders progress', *Care Plan*, vol 6, no 4, pp 17–20.

Brindle, D. (2008) 'Tireless champion of autonomy', *Guardian Society*, 22 October, available online via www.guardiansociety.co.uk (accessed 24/10/2008).

Brown, G. (2008) 'Speech on the National Health Service', 7 January, London, King's College London/Florence Nightingale School of Nursing.

Browne, L. (1990) *Survey of local authorities direct payments*, London: RADAR.

Browning, D. (2007) *Evaluation of the self-directed support network: a review of progress up to 31st March 2007*, London: Care Services Improvement Partnership.

Burrows, G. (2001) 'Charities criticise draft home care standards', *Community Care*, 21–27 June, p 3.

Butcher, T. (2002) *Delivering welfare* (2nd edn), Buckingham: Open University Press.

Butt, J. and Box, L. (1997) *Supportive services, effective strategies: the views of black-led organisations and social care agencies on the future of social care for black communities*, London: Race Equalities Unit.

Butt, J. et al (eds) (2000) *Directing support: report from a workshop on direct payments and black and minority ethnic disabled people*, York: JRF.

Cabinet Office (2012) *Not-for-profit advice services in England*, London: Cabinet Office.

Campbell, J. (nd) 'Promoting personal assistance to enable independent living', Social Services Conference, 29 October, London: National Centre for Independent Living.

Campbell, J. (1996) 'Implementing direct payments: towards the next millennium', National Institute of Social Work Conference, 12 November.

Carers UK (2008) *Choice or chore? Carers' experiences of direct payments*, London: Carers UK.

Carlin, J. and Lenehan, C. (2004) *Direct experience: a guide for councils on the implementation of direct payments in children's services*, London: Council for Disabled Children.

Carlin, J. and Lenehan, C. (2006) 'Overcoming barriers to the take-up of direct payments by parents of disabled children', in J. Leece and J. Bornat (eds) *Developments in direct payments*, Bristol: The Policy Press.

Carmichael, A. and Brown, L. (2002) 'The future challenge for direct payments', *Disability and Society*, vol 17, no 7, pp 797–808.

Carr, S. (2010) *Enabling risk, ensuring safety: self-directed support and personal budgets*, London: SCIE.

Carr, S. (2011) 'Enabling risk and ensuring safety: self-directed support and personal budgets', *Journal of Adult Protection*, vol 13, no 3, pp 122–36.

Carr, S. and Robbins, D. (2009) *The implementation of individual budget schemes in adult social care*, London: SCIE.

Chinn, C. (1995) *Poverty amidst prosperity: the urban poor in England, 1834–1914*, Manchester: Manchester University Press.

CIPFA (Chartered Institute of Public Finance and Accountancy) (1998) *Community care direct payments: accounting and financial management guidelines*, London: CIPFA.

CIPFA (2007) *Direct payments and individual budgets: managing the finances*, London: CIPFA (supported by In Control and the Department of Health).

Clark, H. and Spafford, H. (2002) 'Adapting to the culture of user control?', *Social Work Education*, vol 21, no 2, pp 247–57.

Clark, H. et al (1998) *That bit of help: the high value of low level preventative services for older people*, Bristol/York: The Policy Press/JRF.

Clark, H. et al (2004) *'It pays dividends': direct payments and older people*, Bristol: The Policy Press.

Commission for Rural Communities (2008) *Tailor made? The implications of the personalisation of social care for older people living in rural communities*, London: Commission for Rural Communities.

Conservative Party (2007) *NHS autonomy and accountability: proposals for legislation*, London: Conservative Party.

Craig, G. (1992) *Cash or care: a question of choice? Cash, community care and user participation*, York: Social Policy Research Unit, University of York.

Crosby, N. (2008) 'Children and families in control', in C. Hatton et al *A report on In Control's second phase: evaluation and learning 2005–2007*, London: In Control Publications.

CSCI (Commission for Social Care Inspection) (2004) *Direct payments: what are the barriers?*, London: CSCI.

CSCI (2006) *Time to care? An overview of home care services for older people in England, 2006*, London: CSCI.

CSCI (2008a) *State of social care in England 2006–07*, London: CSCI.

CSCI (2008b) *Putting people first: equality and diversity matters 1 – providing appropriate services for lesbian, gay and bisexual and transgender people*, London: CSCI.

CSIP (Care Services Improvement Partnership) (2008) 'Micro markets project: report on progress after one year', available online via http://individualbudgets. csip.org.uk (accessed 29/08/2008).

Da Roit and Le Bihan (2010) 'Similar and yet so different: cash-for-care in six European countries' long-term care policies', *The Milbank Quarterly*, vol 88, no 3, pp 286–309.

Daly, G. and Roebuck, A. (2008) 'Gaining independence: an evaluation of service users' accounts of the individual budgets pilots', *Journal of Integrated Care*, vol 16, no 3, pp 17–25.

Darzi, A. (2008) *High quality care for all: NHS next stage review final report* (Darzi Report), London: The Stationery Office (TSO).

Davey, V. et al (2007a) *Schemes providing support to people using direct payments: a UK survey*, London: Personal Social Services Research Unit, London School of Economics and Political Science.

Davey, V. et al (2007b) *Direct payments: a national survey of direct payments policy and practice*, London: Personal Social Services Research Unit, London School of Economics and Political Science.

Davidson, D. and Luckhurst, L. (2002) *Making choices, taking control: direct payments and mental health service users/survivors*, London: National Centre for Independent Living/JRF.

Davis, A. et al (1997) *Access to assessment: perspectives of practitioners, disabled people and carers*, Bristol: The Policy Press.

Dawson, C. (2000) *Independent successes: implementing direct payments*, York: JRF.

DCLG (Department for Communities and Local Government) (2010) 'Councils' red tape cut as 4,700 Whitehall targets slashed', 14 October, available online via https://www.gov.uk/government/news/councils-red-tape-cut-as-4–700-whitehall-targets-slashed (accessed 30/04/2015).

Department for Education (2012) *Special educational needs support: families to be given personal budgets* (press release, 15/05/2012), London: Department for Education.

DH (Department of Health) (1989) *Caring for people: community care in the next decade and beyond*, London: HMSO.

DH (1990) *Community care in the next decade and beyond: policy guidance*, London: DH.

DH (1994) 'Virginia Bottomley gives direct payments to disabled people the go ahead', 24 November, press release 94/537, London: DH.

DH (1997) *Community Care (Direct Payments) Act 1996: policy and practice guidance*, London: DH.

DH (1998a) *Independence pays: Community Care (Direct Payments) Act 1996*, DH information video, London: DH.

DH (1998b) *Modernising social services: promoting independence, improving protection, raising standards*, London: TSO.

DH (2000) *Community Care (Direct Payments) Act 1996: policy and practice guidance* (2nd edn), London: DH.

DH (2001a) *Carers and Disabled Children Act 2000: carers and people with parental responsibility for disabled children – practice guidance*, London: DH.

DH (2001b) *Carers and Disabled Children Act 2000: carers and people with parental responsibility for disabled children – policy guidance*, London: DH.

DH (2001c) *Carers and Disabled Children Act 2000: direct payments for young disabled people – policy guidance and practice guidance*, London: DH.

DH (2001d) *A practitioner's guide to carers' assessments under the Carers and Disabled Children Act 2000*, London: DH.

DH (2001e) *Explanatory notes to Health and Social Care Act 2001*, available online via www.opsi.gov.uk/Acts/acts2001/en/ukpgaen_20010015_en_1 (accessed 19/06/2001).

DH (2001f) *Valuing people: a new strategy for learning disability for the 21st century*, London: DH.

DH (2003a) *Direct payments guidance: community care, services for carers and children's services (direct payments) guidance, England*, London: DH.

DH (2003b) *Social services performance assessment framework indicators 2002–2003*, London: DH.

DH (2004a) *Direct choices – what councils need to make direct payments happen for people with learning disabilities*, London: DH.

DH (2004b) *An easy guide to direct payments*, London: DH.

DH (2005) *Independence, well-being and choice*, London: TSO.

DH (2006) *Our health, our care, our say*, London: TSO.

DH (2007) *Direct payments uptake project: an easy words leaflet*, London: DH.

DH (2008a) *Transforming social care*, local authority circular LAC(DH)(2008)1.

DH (2008b) *Moving forward: using the learning from the individual budget pilots*, London: DH.

DH (2008c) *Making personal budgets work for older people: developing experience*, London: DH.

DH (2008d) *Putting people first – working to make it happen: adult social care workforce strategy – interim statement*, London: DH.

DH (2009) *Guidance on direct payments – for community care, services for carers and children's services: England*, London: DH.

DH (2010a) *A vision for adult social care: capable communities and active citizens*, London: DH.

DH (2010b) *Putting people first: personal budgets for older people – making it happen*, London: DH.

DH (2011a) *Patients to have a greater say and choice over their care*, DH press release (04/10/2011).

DH (2011b) *Working for personalised care: a framework for supporting personal assistants working in adult social care*, London: DH.

DH (2014a) *Care and support statutory guidance, issued under the Care Act 2014*, London: DH.

DH (2014b) *The mandate: a mandate from the government to NHS England, April 2015 to March 2016*, London: DH.

DH and the Right Hon Norman Lamb (2014) *Care Bill becomes Care Act 2014*, available online via www.gov.uk/government/speeches/care-bill-becomes-care-act-2014 (accessed 07/05/2015).

DH/Care Services Improvement Partnership/In Control (2008) *Individual budgets: living your life, your way*, DH DVD.

DH/Scottish Office/Welsh Office/Northern Ireland Office (1996) *Community Care (Direct Payments) Bill: consultation paper*, London: DH.

DH/SSI (Social Services Inspectorate) (1996) *Progressing services with physically disabled people: report on inspections of community services for physically disabled people*, London: DH.

DH/SSI (1997) *Inspection of community care services for black and minority ethnic older people: Birmingham*, Nottingham: Central Inspection Group, SSI.

DH/SSI (1999a) *Inspection of independent living arrangements for younger disabled people: Poole Borough Council*, Bristol: South and West Inspection Group, SSI.

DH/SSI (1999b) *Inspection of independent living arrangements for younger disabled people: Middlesbrough Borough Council*, Gateshead: North East Inspection Group, SSI.

DH/SSI (1999c) *Inspection of independent living arrangements for younger disabled people: County of Herefordshire District Council*, Bristol: South and West Inspection Group, SSI.

DHSS (Department of Health and Social Security) (1981) *Growing older*, London: HMSO.

DHSSPS (Department of Health, Social Services and Public Safety) (1997) *Personal Social Services (Direct Payments) (Northern Ireland) Order 1996: guidance for boards and trusts*, Belfast: DHSSPS.

DHSSPS (2000a) *A guide to receiving direct payments*, Belfast: TSO.

DHSSPS (2000b) *Personal Social Services (Direct Payments) (Northern Ireland) Order 1996: guidance for boards and trusts*, Belfast: DHSSPS.

DHSSPS (2004) *Direct payments legislation and guidance for boards and trusts*, Belfast: DHSSPS.

Dickens, C. (1867) *Oliver Twist*, London: Chapman and Hall.

Dickie, E. (2013) *A personalised approach to prison resettlement: lessons from a pilot project*, London: Revolving Doors.

Donovan, T. (2014) 'Preparing for life after the Independent Living Fund', *Community Care,* 14 March, available online via www.communitycare. co.uk/2014/03/14/preparing-life-independent-living-fund/ (accessed 13/04/2015).

Dowson, S. (2002) *Not just about the money: reshaping social care for social determination*, Stockport: Community Living and Emprise International Training and Consultancy.

Duffy, S. (2004) 'In Control', *Journal of Integrated Care*, vol 12, no 6, pp 7–13.

Duffy, S. (2005a) 'Individual budgets: Transforming the allocation of resources for care', *Journal of Integrated Care*, vol 13, no 1, pp 8-16.

Duffy, S. (2005b) 'Will 'in Control' at last put people in charge of their lives?', *Community Living*, vol 18, no 4, pp 10-13.

Duffy, S. (2005c) *Keys to citizenship: a guide to getting good support for people with learning disabilities* (re-printed from 2003 edition, with additional new chapter), Birkenhead: Paradigm.

Duffy, S. (2006) 'The implications of individual budgets', *Journal of Integrated Care*, vol 14, no 2, pp 3–10.

Duffy, S. (2007) 'Care management and self-directed support', *Journal of Integrated Care*, vol 15, no 5, pp 3–14.

Duffy, S. (2008) 'Self-directed support is for everyone', in C. Hatton et al *A report on In Control's second phase: evaluation and learning 2005–2007*, London: In Control Publications.

Duffy, S. (2010) *A fair income: tax-benefit reform in an era of personalisation*, Sheffield/Birmingham: Centre for Welfare Reform/Health Services Management Centre.

Duffy, S. (2012a) *Is personalisation dead?*, available online via www.centreforwelfarereform.org/library/by-date/is-personalisation-dead.html (accessed 22/05/2015).

Duffy, S. (2012b) *An apology*, available online via www.centreforwelfarereform.org/library/type/text/an-apology.html (accessed 22/05/2015).

Duffy, S. (2013) *A fair society? How the cuts target disabled people*, Sheffield: the Centre for Welfare Reform (on behalf of the Campaign for a Fair Society).

Duffy, S. (2014) 'After personalisation', in C. Needham and J. Glasby (eds) (2014) *Debates in personalisation*, Bristol: The Policy Press.

Duffy, S. and Waters, J. (2008) 'The economics of self-directed support', in C. Hatton et al *A report on In Control's second phase: evaluation and learning 2005–2007*, London: In Control Publications.

Dunnicliff, J. (1999) *Funding for personal assistance support services: the key to making personal assistance schemes work*, London: NCIL.

DWP (Department for Work and Pensions) (2005) *Opportunity age: meeting the challenges of ageing in the 21st century*, London: DWP.

DWP (2014) *Closure of Independent Living Fund (ILF)*, DWP, available via https://www.gov.uk/government/uploads/system/uploads/attachment_data/file/287236/closure-of-ilf-equality-analysis.pdf (accessed 13/04/2015).

Edsall, N.C. (1971) *The anti-Poor Law movement, 1834–1844*, Manchester: Manchester University Press.

Ellis, K. (2005) 'Disability rights in practice: the relationship between human rights and social rights in contemporary social care', *Disability and Society*, vol 20, no 7, pp 691–704.

Ellis, K. (2007) 'Direct payments and social work practice: the significance of "street-level bureaucracy" in determining eligibility', *British Journal of Social Work*, vol 37, pp 405–22.

Ellis, K. et al (1999) 'Needs assessment, street-level bureaucracy and the new community care', *Social Policy and Administration*, vol 33, no 3, pp 262–80.

Ellis Paine, A. et al (2014) *Maximising older people's personal budget use (MOPPU): project evaluation report*, Birmingham: University of Birmingham/Age UK.

Englander, D. (1998) *Poverty and Poor Law reform in 19th century Britain, 1834–1914: from Chadwick to Booth*, London: Longman.

Ettelt, S. et al (2013) *Trailblazer programme evaluation: preliminary report*, available online via www.piru.ac.uk/assets/files/DP%20Trailblazer%20Preliminary%20report.pdf (accessed 07/05/2015).

Ettelt, S. et al (2015) *Evaluation of direct payments in residential care trailblazers: interim report*, available online via www.piru.ac.uk/assets/files/DPs%20in%20 Residential%20Care%20Trailblazers%20-%20Interim%20Report.pdf (accessed 07/05/2015).

Evans, J. (1993) 'The role of centres of independent/integrated living and networks of disabled people', in C. Barnes (ed) *Making our own choices: independent living, personal assistance and disabled people*, Belper: British Council of Disabled People.

Evans, J. (2000) 'Direct payments in the United Kingdom', presentation at the International Conference on Self-Determination and Individualised Funding, Seattle, 29–31 July.

Evans, J. and Hasler, F. (1996) 'Direct payments campaign in the UK', presentation for the European Network on Independent Living Seminar, Stockholm, 9–11 June.

Ferguson, I. (2007) 'Increasing user choice or privatizing risk? The antimonies of personalization', *British Journal of Social Work*, vol 37, pp 387–403.

Fernandez, J.L. et al (2007) 'Direct payments in England: factors linked to variations in local provision', *Journal of Social Policy*, vol 36, no 1, pp 97–121.

Fletcher, M. (2006) 'Carers and direct payments', in J. Leece and J. Bornat (eds) *Developments in direct payments*, Bristol: The Policy Press.

Forder, J. et al (2012) *Evaluation of the personal health budget pilot programme*, London: DH.

Fraser, D. (1984) *The evolution of the British welfare state* (2nd edn), Basingstoke: Macmillan.

Friedman, M. (1962) *Capitalism and freedom*, Chicago: University of Chicago Press.

Fruin, D. (1998) *Moving into the mainstream: the report of a national inspection of services for adults with learning disabilities*, London: DH.

Fruin, D. (2000) *New directions for independent living*, London: DH.

Fryer, R. (1998) *Signposts to services: inspection of social services information to the public*, London: DH.

Gadsby, E. et al (2013) 'Personal budgets, choice and health: a review of international evidence from 11 OECD countries', *International Journal of Public and Private Healthcare Management and Economics*, vol 3, no 3–4, pp 15–28.

Gainsbury, S. (2008) 'Councils could lose £7bn social care funds to DWP', *Health Service Journal*, 29 May, available online via www.hsj.co.uk (accessed 07/07/2008).

Gardner, A. (1999) *Making direct payments a reality for people with learning difficulties*, Whalley: North West Training and Development Team.

Gardner, A. (2014) *Personalisation in social work* (2nd edn), London: Sage.

George, M. (1994) 'Flexible choices', *Community Care*, 24–30 November, pp 14–15.

George, M. (1996) 'Cash on the nail', *Community Care*, 17–23 October, pp 24–5.

George, M. (2001) 'Our way or no way', *Community Care*, 12–18 July, pp 32–3.

Gillespie, J. with Hughes, S. (2010) *Positively local: C2 – a model for community change*, Sheffield/Birmingham: Centre for Welfare Reform/Health Services Management Centre.

Glasby, J. (2008) *Individual budgets and the interface with health: a discussion paper for the Care Services Improvement Partnership*, Birmingham: Health Services Management Centre.

Glasby, J. (2011) *Whose risk is it anyway? Risk and regulation in an era of personalisation* (JRF scoping paper), York: JRF.

Glasby, J. (2012a) *Understanding health and social care* (2nd edn) Bristol: The Policy Press.

Glasby, J. (2012b) 'Whose risk is it anyway? Risk and regulation in an era of personalisation', *Journal of Care Services Management*, vol 5, no 4, pp 173–83.

Glasby, J. and Beresford, P. (2006) 'Who knows best? Evidence-based practice and the service user contribution', *Critical Social Policy*, vol 26, no 1, pp 268–84.

Glasby, J. and Duffy, S. (2007) *'Our Health, Our Care, Our Say' – what could the NHS learn from individual budgets and direct payments?*, Birmingham: Health Services Management Centre/In Control.

Glasby, J. and Hasler, F. (2004) *A healthy option? Direct payments and the implications for health care*, Birmingham: Health Services Management Centre/National Centre for Independent Living.

Glasby, J. and Littlechild, R. (2004) *The health and social care divide: the experiences of older people* (2nd edn), Bristol: The Policy Press.

Glasby, J. et al (eds) (2007) 'Evidence-based practice', special edition of *Evidence and Policy*, vol 3, no 3, pp 323–457.

Glendinning, C. (2010) 'Reforming adult social care: what can England learn from the experiences of other countries', *Quality in Ageing and Older Adults*, vol 11, no 4, pp 40–6.

Glendinning, C. and Kemp, P. (eds) (2006) *Cash and care: policy challenges in the welfare state*, Bristol: The Policy Press.

Glendinning, C. et al (2000a) *Buying independence: using direct payments to integrate health and social services*, Bristol: The Policy Press.

Glendinning, C. et al (2000b) 'Bridging the gap: using direct payments to purchase integrated care', *Health and Social Care in the Community*, vol 8, no 3, pp 192–200.

Glendinning, C. et al (2000c) 'New kinds of care, new kinds of relationships: how purchasing services affects relationships in giving and receiving personal assistance', *Health and Social Care in the Community*, vol 8, no 3, pp 201–11.

Glendinning, C. et al (2008) *Evaluation of the individual budgets pilot programme*, York: Social Policy Research Unit.

Glendinning, C. et al (2009) *The individual budgets pilot projects: impact and outcomes for carers*, York: Social Policy Research Unit.

Glendinning, C. et al (2015) 'Ambiguity in practice? Carers' roles in personalised social care in England', *Health and Social Care in the Community*, vol 23, no 1, pp 23–32.

Glynn, M. et al (2008) *Person-centred support: what service users and practitioners say*, York: JRF.

Grasser, G. et al (2013) 'Personal health budgets in the Netherlands and England', *Eurohealth*, vol 19, no 2, pp 21–23.

Greenwood, W. (1969) *Love on the dole*, Harmondsworth: Penguin.

Grimshaw, J. and Fletcher, S. (nd) *Direct payments: people with HIV – the way forward*, London: National AIDS Trust/National Centre for Independent Living.

Harding, M.L. (2005) 'Patients could get their own budgets, Number 10 says', *Health Service Journal*, 18 May, available online via www.hsj.co.uk (accessed 02/12/2008).

Hasler, F. (1997) 'Living is about more than bed and breakfast', *Health Matters*, vol 32, pp 12–13.

Hasler, F. (1999) 'Exercising the right to freedom of choice', *Professional Social Work*, June, pp 6–7.

Hasler, F. (2000) 'What is direct payments', in J. Butt et al (eds) *Directing support: report from a workshop on direct payments and black and minority ethnic disabled people*, York: JRF.

Hasler, F. (2006) 'The Direct Payments Development Fund', in J. Leece and J. Bornat (eds) *Developments in direct payments*, Bristol: The Policy Press.

Hasler, F. and Marshall, S. (2013) *Trust is the key: increasing the take-up of direct payments*, London: Disability Rights UK.

Hasler, F. et al (1998) *Key issues for local authority implementation of direct payments* (first published 1998, revised 1999), available online via www.psi.org.uk/publications/DISAB/key%20issues.htm (accessed 18/01/2001).

Hasler, F. et al (1999) *Direct routes to independence: a guide to local authority implementation and management of direct payments*, London: Policy Studies Institute.

Hatchett, W. (1991) 'Cash on delivery?', *Community Care*, 30 May, pp 14–15.

Hatton, C. et al (2008) *A report on In Control's second phase: evaluation and learning 2005–2007*, London: In Control Publications.

Hatton, C. (2015) 'Independent living – a charismatic, chameleonic or institutional idea?', available online via https://theindependentlivingdebate.wordpress.com/2014/04/15/independent-living-a-charismatic-chameleonic-or-institutional-idea/ (accessed 18/06/2015).

Hayek, F. (1944) *The road to serfdom*, London: Routledge and Kegan Paul.

Health Foundation (2010) *Personal health budgets: research scan*, London: Health Foundation.

Health Foundation (2011) *The personal touch: the Dutch experience of personal health budgets*, London: Health Foundation.

Health and Social Care Board (2015) *Draft equality impact assessment on self-directed support*, Belfast: Health and Social Care Board.

Help the Aged (2002) *Direct payments, direct control: enabling older people to manage their own care*, London: Help the Aged.

Henwood, M. and Hudson, B. (2007a) *Review of the Independent Living Funds*, London: Department for Work and Pensions.

Henwood, M. and Hudson, B. (2007b) *Here to stay? Self-directed support: aspiration and implementation (a review for the Department of Health)*, Heathencote: Melanie Henwood Associates.

Henwood, M. and Hudson, B. (2009) *Keeping it personal: supporting people with multiple and complex needs – a report to the Commission for Social Care Inspection*, Heathencote: Melanie Henwood Associates.

Heslop, P. (2001) 'Direct payments for people with mental health support needs', *The Advocate*, May, pp 8–9.

Hirst, J. (1997) 'Direct benefit?', *Community Care*, 1 May, pp 10–11.

HM Government (2007) *Putting people first: a shared vision and commitment to the transformation of adult social care*, London: HM Government.

HM Government (2012) *Caring for our future: reforming care and support*, London: TSO.

Holman, A. and Bewley, C. (1999) *Funding freedom 2000: people with learning difficulties using direct payments*, London: Values into Action.

Hough, J. and Rice, B. (2010) *Providing personalised support to rough sleepers*, York: JRF.

House of Commons Health Committee (1993) *Community care: the way forward – volume I* (Sixth Report), London: HMSO.

HSCIC (Health and Social Care Information Centre) (2014) *Community care statistics: social services activity, England*, London: HSCIC.

Hudson, B. (1988) 'Doomed from the start?', *Health Service Journal*, 23 June, pp 708–9.

Hudson, B. (1993) 'The Icarus effect', *Health Service Journal*, 18 November, pp 27–9.

Hudson, B. (1994) 'Independent living for people in Britain: too successful by half? The case of the Independent Living Fund', *Critical Social Policy*, vol 40, pp 88–96.

Hutchinson, P. et al (2006) 'North American approaches to individualised planning and direct funding', in J. Leece and J. Bornat (eds) *Developments in direct payments*, Bristol: The Policy Press.

Hyde, C. (2010) *Local justice: family-focused reinvestment*, Sheffield/Birmingham: Centre for Welfare Reform/Health Services Management Centre.

IFF Research (2008) *Employment aspects and workforce implications of direct payments*, London: IFF Research.

ILF (Independent Living Fund) (2000) *Guidance notes for the 93 Fund and Extension Fund*, Nottingham: ILF.

Jones, R. (2000) *Getting going on direct payments*, Trowbridge: Wiltshire Social Services, on behalf of the Association of Directors of Social Services.

Jordan, B. (1974) *Poor parents: social policy and the 'cycle of deprivation'*, London: Routledge and Kegan Paul.

Kestenbaum, A. (1993a) *Making community care a reality: the Independent Living Fund, 1988–1993*, London: RADAR.

Kestenbaum, A. (1993b) *Cash for care: a report on the experience of Independent Living Fund clients* (2nd edn), London: RADAR/Disablement Income Group.

Kestenbaum, A. (1999) *What price independence? Independent living and people with high support needs*, Bristol/York: The Policy Press/JRF.

Killin, D. (1993) 'Independent living, personal assistance, disabled lesbians and gay men', in C. Barnes (ed) *Making our own choices: independent living, personal assistance and disabled people*, Belper: British Council of Disabled People.

Kinnaird, L. and Fearnley, K. (2010) *Let's get personal – personalisation and dementia*, Edinburgh: Alhzeimer Scotland.

Kobasa, S. (1979) 'Stressful life events, personality and health: an inquiry into hardiness', *Journal of Personality and Social Psychology*, vol 37, no 1, pp 1–11.

Labour Party (2005) *The Labour Party 2005 manifesto: Britain forwards, not back*, London: Labour Party.

Lakey, J. (1994) *Caring about independence: disabled people and the Independent Living Fund*, London: Policy Studies Institute.

Lakey, L. and Saunders, T. (2011) *Getting personal? Making personal budgets work for people with dementia*, London: Alzheimer's Society.

Larsen, J. et al (2013) 'Implementing personalisation for people with mental health problems: a comparative case study of four local authorities in England', *Journal of Mental Health*, vol 22, no 2, pp 174–82.

Law Commission (2011) *Adult social care (presented to Parliament pursuant to section 3(2) of the Law Commissions Act 1965)*, London: TSO.

Laybourne, A.H. et al (2014) 'Beginning to explore the experience of managing a direct payment for someone with dementia: the perspectives of suitable people and adult social care practitioners', *Dementia*, doi: 10.1177/1471301214553037.

Leadbeater, C., Bartlett, J. and Gallagher, N. (2008) *Making it personal*, London: Demos.

Leece, D. and Leece, J. (2006) 'Direct payments: creating a two-tiered system in social care?', *British Journal of Social Work*, vol 36, pp 1379–93.

Leece, J. (2000) 'It's a matter of choice: making direct payments work in Staffordshire', *Practice*, vol 12, no 4, pp 37–48.

Leece, J. (2002) 'Extending direct payments to informal carers: some issues for local authorities', *Practice*, vol 14, no 2, pp 31–44.

Leece, J. (2003) *Direct payments*, Birmingham: Venture Press.

Leece, J. (2004) 'Money talks but what does it say? Direct payments and the commodification of care', *Practice*, vol 16, no 3, pp 211–21.

Leece, J. (2006a) 'Direct payments and user-controlled support: the challenges for social care commissioning', *Practice*, vol 19, no 3, pp 185–98.

Leece, J. (2006b) '"It's not like being at work": a study to investigate stress and job satisfaction in employees of direct payment users', in J. Leece and J. Bornat (eds) *Developments in direct payments*, Bristol: The Policy Press.

Leece, J. (2010) 'Paying the piper and calling the tune: power and the direct payment relationship', *British Journal of Social Work*, vol 40, no 1, pp 188–206.

Leece, J. and Bornat, J. (eds) (2006) *Developments in direct payments*, Bristol: The Policy Press.

Le Grand, J. (2007) *The other invisible hand: delivering public services through choice and competition*, Princeton: Princeton University Press.

Lewis, J. (1995) *The voluntary sector, the state and social work in Britain*, Aldershot: Edward Elgar.

Lewis, J. (1996) 'What does contracting do to voluntary agencies?', in D. Billis and M. Harris (eds) *Voluntary agencies: challenges of organisations and management*, Basingstoke: Macmillan.

Lindblom, C. (1959) 'The science of muddling through', *Public Administration Review*, vol 19, no 2, pp 78–88.

Lipsky, M. (1980) *Street-level bureaucracy: dilemmas of the individual in public services*, New York: Russell Sage Foundation.

Littlechild, R. et al (2011) 'Risk and personalisation', in H. Kemshall and B. Wilkinson (eds) *Good practice in assessing risk: current knowledge, issues and approaches*, London: Jessica Kingsley.

Lombard, D. (2008) 'Self-directed care schemes in Scotland break employment law', *Community Care*, 17 June.

Lombard, D. (2009) 'Wales at odds with England over personal budgets', *Community Care*, 19 June, available online via www.communitycare.co.uk/2009/06/19/wales-at-odds-with-england-over-personal-budgets/.

Lord, P. and Hutchinson, P. (2003) 'Individualised support and funding: building blocks for capacity building and inclusion', *Disability and Society*, vol 18, no 1, pp 71–86.

Lundsgaard, J. (2005) *Consumer direction and choice in long-term care for older persons, including payments for informal care: how can it help improve care outcomes, employment and fiscal sustainability?* OECD Health Working Paper no 20, Paris: OECD.

Macfarlane, A. (1990) 'The right to make choices', *Community Care*, 1 November, pp 14–15.

Maglajlic, R. (1999) 'The silent treatment', *Openmind*, September/October, pp 12–13.

Maglajlic, R. et al (1998) 'Direct payments in mental health – a research report', *Breakthrough*, vol 2, no 3, pp 33–43.

Maglajlic, R. et al (2000) 'Making direct payments a choice: a report on the research findings', *Disability & Society*, vol 15, no 1, pp 99–113.

Mandelstam, M. (1999) *Community care practice and the law* (2nd edn), London: Jessica Kingsley.

Manthorpe, J. and Samsi, K. (2013) '"Inherently risky?": personal budgets for people with dementia and the risks of financial abuse: findings from an interview-based study with adult safeguarding coordinators', *British Journal of Social Work*, vol 43, no 5, pp 889–903.

Manthorpe, J. et al (2009a) 'Training for change: early days of individual budgets and the implications for social work and care management practice', *British Journal of Social Work*, vol 39, no 7, pp 1291–305.

Manthorpe, J. et al (2009b) 'Safeguarding and system change: early perceptions of the implications for adult protection services of the English individual budgets pilots – a qualitative study', *British Journal of Social Work*, vol 39, no 8, pp 1465–80.

Manthorpe, J. et al (2010) 'Individual budgets and adult safeguarding: parallel or converging tracks? Further findings from the evaluation of the individual budget pilots', *Journal of Social Work*, vol 11, no 4, 422–38.

Manthorpe, J. et al (2011a) 'Keeping it in the family? People with learning disabilities employing their own care and support workers: findings from a scoping review of the literature', *Journal of Intellectual Disabilities*, vol 15, no 3, pp 195–207.

Manthorpe, J. et al (2011b) *Self-directed support: a review of the barriers and facilitators*, Edinburgh: Scottish Government Social Research.

Manthorpe, J. et al (2015a) 'Embarking on self-directed support in Scotland: a focused scoping review of the literature', *European Journal of Social Work*, vol 18, no 1, pp 36–50.

Manthorpe, J. et al (2015b) 'Did anyone notice the transformation of adult social care? An analysis of Safeguarding Adult Board Annual Reports', *Journal of Adult Protection*, vol 17, no 1, pp 19–30.

Mantle, G. and Backwith, D. (2010) 'Poverty and social work', *British Journal of Social Work*, vol 40, pp 2380–97.

Marchant, R. et al (2007) *'Necessary stuff' – the social care needs of children with complex health care needs and their families*, London: SCIE.

McCurry, P. (1999) 'The direct route', *Community Care*, 9–15 September, pp 20–1.

McKay, S. and Rowlingson, K. (1999) *Social security in Britain*, Basingstoke: Macmillan.

McMullen, M. (2003) *The direct approach*, London: SCOPE.

Means, R. and Smith, R. (1998a) *Community care: policy and practice* (2nd edn), Basingstoke: Macmillan.

Means, R. and Smith, R. (1998b) *From Poor Law to community care: the development of welfare services for elderly people, 1939–1971* (2nd edn), Bristol: The Policy Press.

Means, R. et al (2008) *Community care: policy and practice* (4th edn), Bristol: The Policy Press.

Mental Health Foundation (2011) *Personalisation and dementia: a practitioner's guide to self-directed support for people living with dementia*, London: Mental Health Foundation.

Mickel, A. (2008) 'What's the outlook for adult care?', *Community Care*, 23 October, pp 28–30.

Milburn, A. (2007) 'A 2020 vision for public services', speech at the London School of Economics, 16 May.

Mitchell, W. et al (2015) *Taking on and taking over: choice and control for physically disabled young adults*, SSRC Research Findings, London: NIHR School for Social Care Research.

Moffatt, S. et al (2012) 'Choice, consumerism and devolution: growing old in the welfare state(s) of Scotland, Wales and England', *Ageing and Society*, vol 32, no 5, pp 725–46.

Moore, D. and Nicol, T. (2009) *Getting a blue life: personalisation and the criminal justice system*, Yorkshire and Humber Improvement Partnership.

Moran, N. et al (2011) 'Joining up government by integrating funding streams? The experiences of the Individual Budget Pilot Projects for older and disabled people in England', *International Journal of Public Administration*, vol 34, no 4, pp 232–43.

Morris, J. (1993a) *Independent lives: community care and disabled people*, Basingstoke: Macmillan.

Morris, J. (1993b) 'Advocating true reform', *Community Care*, 4 February, pp 16–17.

Morris, J. (1995) 'How to get money to pay for personal assistance and have control over how its spent', in British Council of Disabled People (ed) *Controlling your own personal assistance services*, available online via www.independentliving.org/docs/enilbcodppayschemes2.html (accessed 30/01/2001).

Morris, J. (1997) 'Care or empowerment? A disability rights perspective', *Social Policy and Administration*, vol 31, no 1, pp 54–60.

Morris, J. and Wates, M. (2006) *Supporting disabled parents and parents with additional support needs*, London: SCIE.

Morris, J. and Wates, M. (2007) *Working together to support disabled parents*, London: SCIE.

Murray, C. (1984) *Losing ground: American social policy 1950–1980*, New York: Basic Books.

Murray, P. (2010) *A fair start: a personalised pathway for disabled children and their families*, Sheffield/Birmingham: Centre for Welfare Reform/Health Services Management Centre.

National Assembly for Wales (1997) *Community Care (Direct Payments) Act 1996: policy and practice guidance*, Cardiff: National Assembly for Wales.

National Assembly for Wales (2000) *Community Care (Direct Payments) Act 1996: policy and practice guidance*, Cardiff: National Assembly for Wales.

NCIL (National Centre for Independent Living) (nda) 'Promoting personal assistance to enable independent living', unpublished information sheet, London: NCIL.

NCIL (ndb) *Community Care (Direct Payments) Act 1996 government review: response by the British Council of Disabled People's National Centre for Independent Living*, London: NCIL.

NCIL (ndc) *Response to consultation on CIPFA draft guidance on direct payments*, London: NCIL.

NCIL (1999) *Government White Paper: Modernising social services – response by the British Council of Disabled People's National Centre for Independent Living*, London: NCIL.

NCIL (2000) *NCIL briefing on the Carers and Disabled Children Bill*, London: NCIL.

NCIL (2003) Transcript of speech by Stephen Ladyman, Parliamentary Under Secretary of State, Department of Health, at NCIL launch event, 30 October, London.

NCIL (2006) *The Direct Payments Development Fund*, London: NCIL/DH.

Needham, C. (2010) 'Personalisation: from storyline to practice', *Journal of Social Policy and Administration*, vol 45, no 1, pp 54–68.

Needham, C. (2011) *Personalising public services: understanding the personalisation narrative*, Bristol: The Policy Press.

Needham, C. and Glasby, J. (eds) (2014) *Debates in personalisation*, Bristol: The Policy Press.

Newbigging, K. with Lowe, J. (2005) *Direct payments and mental health: new directions*, Brighton: Pavilion Publishing.

Newbronner, L. et al (2011) *Keeping personal budgets personal: learning from the experiences of older people, people with mental health problems and their carers*, London: SCIE

NHS Confederation (2015) *Personal budgets in mental health: key points on implementation*, London: NHS Confederation.

NHS England (2014) *Integrated personal commissioning prospectus: making a reality of health and social care integration for individuals*, Leeds: NHS England.

NIMHE (National Institute for Mental Health in England) (2006) *Direct payments for people with mental health problems: a guide to action*, London: DH.

Novak, T. (1988) *Poverty and the state: an historical sociology*, Buckingham: Open University Press.

O'Hara, M. (2014) *Austerity bites*, Bristol: The Policy Press.

Oliver, M. (1990) *The politics of disablement*, Basingstoke: Macmillan.

Oliver, M. (1996) *Understanding disability: from theory to practice*, Basingstoke: Macmillan.

Oliver, M. and Sapey, B. (1999) *Social work with disabled people* (2nd edn), Basingstoke: Macmillan.

Oliver, M. and Zarb, G. (1992) *Greenwich personal assistance schemes: second year evaluation*, London: Greenwich Association of Disabled People.

OPM (Office for Public Management) (2006) *Budget-holding lead professionals: literature review – report for the Department for Education and Skills*, London: OPM.

OPM (2007) *The implications of individual budgets for service providers*, London: OPM.

Parrott, L. (2014) *Social work and poverty: a critical approach*, Bristol: The Policy Press.

Payne, M. (2005) *The origins of social work: continuity and change*, Basingstoke: Palgrave.

Pearson, C. (2000) 'Money talks? Competing discourses in the role of direct payments', *Critical Social Policy*, vol 20, no 4, pp 459–77.

Pearson, C. (2004) 'Keeping the cash under control: what's the problem with direct payments in Scotland?', *Disability and Society*, vol 19, no 1, pp 3–14.

Pearson, C. (2006) 'Direct payments in Scotland', in J. Leece and J. Bornat (eds) *Developments in direct payments*, Bristol: The Policy Press.

Pearson, C. et al (2014) *Self-directed support: personalisation, choice and control*, Edinburgh: Dunedin Academic Press.

Pijl, M. (2000) 'Home care allowances: good for many but not for all', *Practice*, vol 12, no 2, pp 55–65.

Pile, H. (2014) 'What about the workforce?', in C. Needham and J. Glasby (eds) *Debates in personalisation*, Bristol: the Policy Press.

Poldervaart, H. and Malenczuk, L. (2013) *Direct payments for social care: options for managing the cash*, London: Age UK.

Poll, C. et al (2006) *A report on In Control's first phase, 2003–2005*, London: In Control Publications.

Poole, T. (2006) *Direct payments and older people* (background paper commissioned by the Wanless Review), London: King's Fund.

Powell, M. (2015) 'Who killed the English National Health Service?', *International Journal of Health Policy and Management*, vol 4, no 5, pp 267–9.

Powell, M. and Miller, R. (2014) 'Framing privatisation in the English National Health Service', *Journal of Social Policy*, vol 43, no 3, pp 575–94.

Prabkahar, M. et al (2011) *Individual budgets for families with disabled children: final evaluation report – the IB process*, London: Department for Education.

Priestley, M. et al (2007) 'Direct payments and disabled people in the UK: supply, demand and devolution', *British Journal of Social Work*, vol 37, pp 1189–204.

Prime Minister's Strategy Unit (2005) *Improving the life chances of disabled people*, London: Prime Minister's Strategy Unit.

Project 81 (nd) *Project 81 – one step up*, Petersfield: HCIL Papers.

Rabiee, P. and Glendinning, C. (2014) 'Choice and control for older people using home care services. How far have council-managed personal budgets helped?', *Quality in Ageing and Older Adults*, vol 15, no 4, pp 210–19.

Rabiee, P. et al (2009) 'Individual budgets: lessons from early users' experience', *British Journal of Social Work*, vol 39, no 5, pp 918–35.

Ratzka, A. (nd) 'What is independent living?', unpublished information sheet, London: NCIL.

Raynes, N. et al (2001) *Quality at home for older people: involving service users in defining home care specifications*, Bristol: The Policy Press/JRF.

Rees, S. (1978) *Social work face to face*, London: Edward Arnold.

Riddell, S. et al (2005) 'The development of direct payments in the UK: implications for social justice', *Social Policy and Society*, vol 4, no 1, pp 75–85.

Riddell, S. et al (2006) *Disabled people and direct payments: a UK comparative study*, Economics and Social Research Council award RES-000-23-0263.

Ridley, J. and Jones, L. (2003) 'Direct what? The untapped potential of direct payments to mental health service users', *Disability and Society*, vol 18, no 5, pp 643–58.

Ridley, J. et al (2011) *Evaluation of self-directed support test sites in Scotland*, Edinburgh: Scottish Government Social Research.

Rodrigues, R. and Glendinning, C. (2014) 'Choice, competition and care – developments in English social care and the impacts on providers and older users of home care services', *Social Policy and Administration*, doi: 10.1111/spol.12099 (accessed 14/04/2015).

Rooff, M. (1972) *One hundred years of family social work: a study of the family welfare society 1869–1969*, London: Michael Joseph.

Rose, M.E. (1988) *The relief of poverty, 1834–1914* (2nd edn), Basingstoke: Macmillan.

Routledge, M. and Carr, S. (2013) *Improving personal budgets for older people: a review – phase one report*, London: TLAP/SCIE.

Routledge, M. et al (2015) *Getting better outcomes. Personal budgets and older people: follow up report*, London: TLAP.

Royal Commission on Long Term Care (1999) *With respect to old age: long term care – rights and responsibilities*, London: TSO.

Rummery, K. (2006) 'Disabled citizens and social exclusion: the role of direct payments', *Policy & Politics*, vol 34, no 4, pp 633–50.

Ryan, T. and Holman, A. (1998a) *Able and willing? Supporting people with learning difficulties to use direct payments*, London: Values Into Action.

Ryan, T. and Holman, A. (1998b) 'Questions of control and consent', *Care Plan*, vol 5, no 2, pp 10–14.

Ryan, T. and Holman, A. (1998c) *Pointers to control: people with learning difficulties using direct payments*, London: Values Into Action.

Samuel, M. (2013) 'Government to trial personal budgets for adoption support', *Community Care*, 3 January, available online via www.communitycare.co.uk (accessed 10/06/2015).

Sanderson, H. and Miller, R. (2014) *The individual services fund handbook: implementing personal budgets in provider organisations*, London: Jessica Kingsley.

Sapey, B. and Pearson, J. (2004) 'Do disabled people need social workers?', *Social Work and Social Sciences Review*, vol 11, no 3, pp 52–70.

Satyamurti, C. (1981) *Occupational survival*, Oxford: Blackwell.

SCIE (Social Care Institute for Excellence) (2007) *Choice, control and individual budgets: emerging themes*, London: SCIE.

SCIE (2008) *Personalisation: a rough guide*, London: SCIE.

SCIE (2012) *Personalisation briefing: implications for personal assistants*, London: SCIE.

Scottish Executive (2000) *Community Care (Direct Payments) Act 1996 – Community Care (Direct Payments) (Scotland) Amendment Regulations 2000, circular no. CCD4/2000*, Edinburgh: Scottish Executive.

Scottish Executive (2001) 'Chisholm announces £530,000 to promote direct payments', Scottish Executive press release SE0940/2001, 06/04/2001, Edinburgh: Scottish Executive.

Scottish Executive (2003) *Direct Payments and Social Work (Scotland) Act 1968: Sections 12B and C: policy and practice guidance*, Edinburgh: Scottish Executive Health Department, Community Care Division.

Scottish Executive (2007) *National guidance on self-directed support*, Edinburgh: Scottish Executive.

Scottish Government (2010) *Self-directed support: a national strategy for Scotland*, Edinburgh: Scottish Government.

Scottish Government (2011) *Self-directed support (direct payments)*, Scotland, 2011, Edinburgh: Scottish Government.

Scottish Government (2014a) *Statutory guidance to accompany the Social Care (Self-directed Support) (Scotland) Act 2013*, Edinburgh: Scottish Government.

Scottish Government (2014b) *Social care services, Scotland, 2014*, Edinburgh: Scottish Government.

Scottish Office (1997) *Community Care (Direct Payments) Act 1996: policy and practice guidance*, Edinburgh: Scottish Office Social Work Services Group.

Scourfield, P. (2005a) 'Implementing the Community Care (Direct Payments) Act: will the supply of personal assistants meet the demand and at what price?', *Journal of Social Policy*, vol 34, no 3, pp 1–20.

Scourfield, P. (2005b) 'Direct payments', *Working with Older People*, vol 9, issue 4, pp 20–3.

Scourfield, P. (2007) 'Social care and the modern citizen: client, consumer, service user, manager and entrepreneur', *British Journal of Social Work*, vol 37, pp 107–22.

Seligman, M.E.P. (1975) *Helplessness: on depression, development and death*, San Francisco, CA: W.H. Freeman.

Senker, J. (2008) 'Enabling people to plan and arrange support', in C. Hatton et al *A report on In Control's second phase: evaluation and learning 2005–2007*, London: In Control Publications.

Shearer, A. (1984) 'Independence is the name of the game', *Voluntary Action*, vol 2, no 3, pp 10–11.

Simpson, F. with Campbell, J. (1996) *Facilitating and supporting independent living: a guide to setting up a personal assistance support scheme*, London: Disablement Income Group.

Skills for Care (2011) *Personalisation and partnership*, Leeds: Skills for Care.

Skills for Care (2012) *Partnerships for personalisation: a practical guide to successful working relationships between individual employers and their personal assistants, carers and support workers*, Leeds: Skills for Care

Slasberg, C. and Hatton, C. (2011) Personalisation: are personal budgets improving outcomes?', *Community Care*, 30 September, available online via www.communitycare.co.uk/articles/30/09/2011/117526/personalisation-are-personal-budgets-improving-outcomes.htm (accessed 11/06/2015).

Slasberg, C. et al (2012a) 'How self-directed support is failing to deliver personal budgets and personalisation', *Research, Policy and Planning*, vol 29, no 3, pp 161–77.

Slasberg, C. et al (2012b) 'Can personal budgets really deliver better outcome for all at no cost? Reviewing the evidence, costs and quality', *Disability & Society*, vol 27, no 7, pp 1029–34.

Slasberg, C. et al (2014) 'Personalization of health care in England: have the wrong lessons been drawn from the personal health budget pilots?', *Journal of Health Services Research and Policy*, vol 19, no 3, pp 183–8.

Smith, K. (2013) *Beyond evidence-based policy in public health: the interplay of ideas*, Basingstoke: Palgrave Macmillan.

Spandler, H. (2004) 'Friend or foe? Towards a critical assessment of direct payments', *Critical Social Policy*, vol 24, no 2, pp 187–209.

Spandler, H. and Vick, N. (2006) 'Opportunities for independent living using direct payments in mental health', *Health and Social Care in the Community*, vol 14, no 2, pp 107–15.

Stainton, T. (2002) 'Taking rights structurally: rights, disability and social worker responses to direct payments', *British Journal of Social Work*, vol 32, pp 751–63.

Stainton, T. (2005) 'Empowerment and the architecture of rights based social policy', *Journal of Intellectual Disabilities*, vol 9, no 4, pp 289–98.

Stainton, T. and Boyce, S. (2004) '"I have got my life back": users' experience of direct payments', *Disability and Society*, vol 19, no 5, pp 443–54.

Stevens, M. et al (2014) *Risk, safeguarding and personal budgets: exploring relationships and identifying good practice*, London: NIHR School for Social Care Research.

Stevens, S. (2008) 'My problem with trade unions', *Community Care*, 2 June.

Stuart, O. (2006) *Will community-based support services make direct payments a viable option for black and minority ethnic service users and carers?*, London: SCIE.

Taylor, N. (2008) 'Obstacles and dilemmas in the delivery of direct payments to service users with poor mental health', *Practice*, vol 20, no 1, pp 43–55.

Taylor, R. (1994) 'Putting the cash upfront', *ADSS News*, November, pp 16–17.

Taylor, R. (1995) *Community Care (Direct Payments) Bill: briefing paper*, Kingston-upon-Thames: ADSS Disabilities Committee.

Taylor, R. (1996a) 'Independent living and direct payments', speech delivered to the ADSS Spring Conference, Cambridge, April.

Taylor, R. (1996b) 'A coherent policy for direct payments', *ADSS News*, vol 5, no 4, p 20.

Taylor, R. (1996c) 'To the beat of a different drum', *Care Plan*, vol 2, no 4, pp 9–10.

Taylor, R. (1997) 'Funding freedom', presentation to the Values Into Action Funding Freedom Conference, 19 March.

Thane, P. (1996) *Foundations of the welfare state* (2nd edn), London: Longman.

TLAP (2011a) *Think local act personal: a sector-wide commitment to moving forward with personalisation and community-based support*, London: TLAP.

TLAP (2011b) *Making it real: marking progress towards personalised, community based support*, London: TLAP.

TLAP (2011c) *Personal budgets: taking stock, moving forwards*, London: TLAP.

Thompson, N. et al (1994) *Dealing with stress*, Basingstoke: Macmillan.

Tu, T. et al (2013) *Evaluation of the Right to Control Trailblazers: synthesis report*, London: HM Government/Office for Disability Issues.

Tyson, A. (nd) *Strategic commissioning and self-directed support*, London: CSIP.

Ungerson, C. (1997) 'Give them the money: is cash a route to empowerment?', *Social Policy and Administration*, vol 31, no 1, pp 45–53.

Ungerson, C. (1999) 'Personal assistants and disabled people: an examination of a hybrid form of work and care', *Work, Employment and Society*, vol 13, no 4, pp 583–600.

Ungerson, C. (2003) 'Commodified care work in European labour markets', *European Societies*, vol 5, no 4, pp 377–96.

Ungerson, C. (2004) 'Whose empowerment and independence? A cross-national perspective on "cash for care" schemes', *Ageing and Society*, vol 24, pp 189–212.

Ungerson, C. (2006) 'Direct payments and the employment relationship: some insight from cross-national research', in J. Leece and J. Bornat (eds) *Developments in direct payments*, Bristol: The Policy Press.

Ungerson, C. and Yeandle, S. (eds) (2007) *Cash for care systems in developed welfare states*, Basingstoke: Palgrave Macmillan.

Valios, N. (1997) 'Direct payments delayed in Ulster', *Community Care*, 24–30 April, p 3.

Vasey, S. (2000) *The rough guide to managing personal assistants*, London: NCIL.

Vevers, S. (2007) 'Carers of disabled children and direct payments', *Community Care*, 6 December.

Vick, N. et al (2006) *An evaluation of the impact of the social care modernisation programme on the implementation of direct payments*, London: Health and Social Care Advisory Service (with University of Central Lancashire and the Foundation for People with Learning Disabilities).

Walker, J. et al (2009) *Budget holding lead professional pilots in multi-agency children's services in England: national evaluation*, London: Department for Children, Schools and Families.

Wanless, D. (2006) *Securing good care for older people: taking a long-term view*, London: King's Fund.

Waters, J. and Duffy, S. (2007) *Individual budgets: report on individual budget integration*, London, In Control Publications.

Waters, J. and Hatton, C. (2014) *Third national personal budget survey*, In Control/ TLAP/Centre for Disability Research.

Webber, M. et al (2014) 'The effectiveness of personal budgets for people with mental health problems: a systematic review', *Journal of Mental Health*, vol 23, no 3, pp 146–55.

Welch, E. et al (2013) *Implementing personal health budgets within substance misuse services* (PSSRU Discussion Paper 2858), Canterbury: PSSRU/DH.

Welch, V. et al (2011) 'Using direct payments to fund short breaks for families with a disabled child', *Child: Care Health and Development*, vol 38, no 6, pp 900–9.

Wellard, S. (1999) 'The costs of control', *Community Care*, 21–27 January, p 23.

Welsh Assembly Government (2004) *Community care, services for carers and children's services (direct payments) guidance, Wales*, Cardiff: Welsh Assembly Government.

Welsh Assembly Government (2011) *Direct payments guidance: community care services for carers and children's services (direct payments) (Wales) Guidance 2011*, Cardiff: Welsh Assembly Government.

Welsh Government (2014) *Implementation of the Social Services and Well-being (Wales) Act 2014*, Cardiff: Welsh Government.

Wilberforce, M. et al (2011) 'Implementing consumer choice in long-term care: the impact of individual budgets on social care providers in England', *Social Policy & Administration*, vol 45, no 5, pp 593–612.

Wilberforce, M. et al (2012) 'Efficiency, choice and control in social care commissioning', *Public Money & Management*, vol 32, no 4, pp 249–56.

Wilberforce, M. et al (2014) 'Revisiting the causes of stress in social work: sources of job demands, control and support in personalised adult social care', *British Journal of Social Work*, vol 44, pp 812–30.

Williams, V. and Holman, A. (2006) 'Direct payments and autonomy: issues for people with learning difficulties', in J. Leece and J. Bornat (eds) *Developments in direct payments*, Bristol: The Policy Press.

Wistow, G. (2015) *Policy process for implementing individual budgets highlights some of the tensions in public policy evaluation*. London School of Economics blog, http://blogs.lse.ac.uk/healthandsocialcare/2015/04/30/policy-process-for-implementing-individual-budgets-highlights-some-of-the-tensions-in-public-policy-evaluation/ (accessed 01/06/2015).

Witcher, S. et al (2000) *Direct payments: the impact on choice and control for disabled people*, Edinburgh: Scottish Executive Central Research Unit.

Woolham, J. (2013) *Are personal budgets always the best way of delivering personalised social care to older people?*, London: NIHR School for Social Care Research.

Woolham, J. and Benton, C. (2012) 'The costs and benefits of personal budgets for older people: evidence from a single local authority', *British Journal of Social Work*, vol 43, no 8, pp 1472–91.

Zamfir, M. (2013) 'Personalisation through personal budgets: its effectiveness for older adults in social care services – findings from an English-based literature review', *Research, Policy and Planning*, vol 30, no 2, pp 77–89.

Zarb, G. (1998) 'What price independence?', paper presented to the 'Shaping our Futures' Conference, London, 5 June.

Zarb, G. (2013) *Personalisation and independent living*, available online via http://disabilityrightsuk.org/sites/default/files/pdf/spectrumoctober2013.pdf (accessed 02/06/2015).

Zarb, G. and Nadash, P. (1994) *Cashing in on independence: Comparing the costs and benefits of cash and services*, London: BCODP.

Zarb, G. and Oliver, M. (1993) *Ageing with a disability: what do you expect after all these years?*, London: University of Greenwich.

Zarb, G. et al (1997) *Implementation and management of direct payment schemes: first findings – summary*, London: PSI.

Index

References to tables/figures/boxes are in *italics*